Intrauterine Devices
and Their Complications

Intrauterine Devices and Their Complications

David A. Edelman, Ph.D.
International Fertility Research Program
Department of Obstetrics and Gynecology
University of North Carolina at Chapel Hill
Chapel Hill, North Carolina

Gary S. Berger, M.D., MSPH, GACOG
Department of Obstetrics and Gynecology
University of North Carolina at Chapel Hill
Chapel Hill, North Carolina

Louis Keith, M.D., FACOG
Department of Obstetrics and Gynecology
Northwestern University Medical School
and Prentice Women's Hospital and Maternity Center
Chicago, Illinois

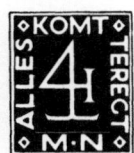

Springer-Science+Business Media, B.V.   1979

Intrauterine Devices and Their Complications

ISBN 978-94-015-0219-1   ISBN 978-94-015-0724-0 (eBook)
DOI 10.1007 /978-94-015-0724-0

The authors and publisher have worked to ensure that all information in this book concerning drug dosages, schedules, and
routes of administration is accurate at the time of publication.
As medical research and practice advance, however, therapeutic
standards may change. For this reason, and because human and
mechanical errors will sometimes occur, we recommend that
our readers consult the *PDR* or a manufacturer's product information sheet prior to prescribing or administering any drug
discussed in this volume.

This book is dedicated to: Nora, Barbara and Gail

Contents

Contents

Foreword

Ever since Hippocrates observed that foreign bodies placed in the uterus would help to prevent pregnancy, periodic interest in this information and its use has resulted in attempts to control unwanted fertility. Prior to the 1900s, this interest was somewhat episodic. Because of anxiety about infection, early attempts flourished only briefly and then were no more. In the twentieth century, however, as a result of renewed interest in intrauterine contraception, particularly in the developing countries, a number of individuals throughout the world began experimenting with a variety of new intrauterine devices. Since then, a great number of these devices have been studied; a few have survived careful scrutiny, and IUDs now represent the second most commonly used form of medical contraception. It is estimated that approximately 15 million devices are in use at the present time, 3 to 4 million of them in the United States.

For a considerable time it was believed that the IUD represented an ideal contraceptive, one defined as totally safe, totally effective, easy to administer, completely reversible, inexpensive and unrelated in its use to the time of sexual intercourse. Unfortunately, the increased use of IUDs and careful study of their effects have proved this original hope to be unfounded.

While still an excellent form of conception control, the IUD does indeed have a number of complications. Over the last decade or two, as innumerable devices have come and gone, their complication rates have varied over a wide range, sparking considerable disagreement concerning the nature, pathogenesis, frequency and treatment of these complications. Much of this confusion was due to the many early studies that were performed using protocols that did not have statistical validity. Data on multiple variables were collected and described in different ways, making it impossible to compare data from one study with another. Moreover, these data were not initially analyzed using the more sophisticated statistical methods, such as the life table technique. Only with the initiation of the Cooperative Statistical Program in 1962 did valid comparative data become available.

The medical literature about intrauterine contraception has grown almost as rapidly as the use of the IUD itself. There now exist innumerable articles on individual devices, chapters in textbooks on contraception and books devoted entirely to the subject. Official documents from the U.S. Food and Drug Administration and a number of health care agencies have also contributed information to the field. Given the current and somewhat confused state of the art and given the increasing relative importance of IUDs as concerns mount about the side effects of oral contraceptives, it is time to publish an analysis of most of the relevant literature to date and to attempt to assess the nature, frequency and treatment of IUD complications.

The authors, drawing on their wide combined experience, have combed the existing literature and drawn together careful evaluations of each of the major complications, pointing out the relevance of the various studies to each issue. Where there are discrepancies in the data and differences of opinion, these are clearly stated. This format allows the reader to draw conclusions, and to realize that in many instances, the final answers remain to be determined.

Intrauterine contraception continues to be of major importance in both developed and developing countries. It is essential to have a book where the various complications are systematically examined, where the issues are defined and where the relevant literature is cited so that further reading on any particular subject is facilitated.

This volume is sufficiently clinical to be of value to those using intrauterine devices in their practice of medicine. It is also sufficiently detailed, well-documented and well-researched to be of value to investigators in the field of intrauterine contraception.

The authors, each an authority in a particular field, are to be congratulated on having taken on a monumental task and having reduced a very complicated segment of the medical literature to such a useful and readable form.

Elizabeth B. Connell, M.D.
May 1979

The IUD, as one of the most effective methods of contraception, has been subject to more highs and lows of professional and public acceptance than has any other method of contraception. The first high was related to initially unrealistic expectations for its performance by health professionals, while the lows have resulted from often inaccurate publicity concerning potential risks and complications associated with its use. Now that significant data have shown most of the potential adverse effects, including even rare events that may occur with its use, it is important that these be placed in correct perspective so that clinicians and users alike may know and understand the risk-benefit ratio associated with IUD use. This book presents the balanced view that all persons involved in the field of contraception need to know. Dissemination of this knowledge will assist health professionals in providing their clients with the information they must have so that the individual woman in consultation with her clinician can make an informed decision as to whether or not the IUD is for her.

Louise B. Tyrer, M.D., FACOG
May 1979

In Memoriam

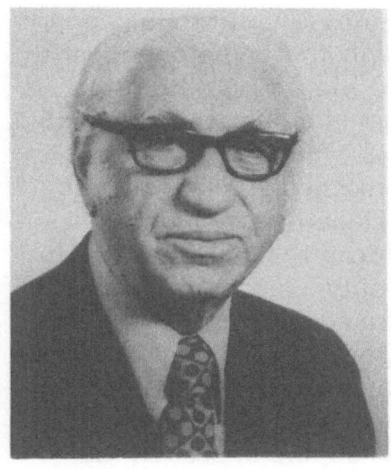

Charles A. Fields, M.D.

Charlie Fields was a beloved friend, a skilled physician and a man of great compassion and commitment. Long before it was fashionable, he dedicated his career to improving the reproductive health of women. A major portion of his professional life was focused on increasing the awareness and availability of safe and effective methods of contraception and abortion, and advancing nurse-midwifery as a profession.

Charlie's commitment to these issues was the result of deep, personal convictions strengthened by understandings gained from his patients and through observation of their lives. Charlie's service at Cook County Hospital and at Mount Sinai Medical Center represented a large and varied patient population which included people from every walk of life and many ethnic backgrounds. As busy and involved as Charlie was, he never limited his practice or compromised the high level of concern and care he felt every patient deserved.

The study of parturition and the forces which came into play at its initiation were the chief focus

of Charlie's academic career. He was particularly
concerned with the development of the lower uterine
segment prior to or at the onset of labor. He often
disagreed with his colleagues regarding this and
other physiological concepts that remain unclear to
this day. Those who heard him present his argu-
ments were always impressed by his vast knowledge
and experience.

His academic career reached a peak when he
accepted the chair of the Department of Obstetrics
and Gynecology at the Chicago Medical School. In
this new role he was not only a leader, but also a
teacher, a confidant and an advisor. As always, he
was sincerely concerned for the welfare of the many
people—students, residents and others—who turned
to him for help or guidance. Charlie was able to
make everyone feel respected and at ease in his
presence and he never considered any problem un-
important or any question foolish. He gained the
respect and admiration of all who knew him.

Shortly after his death in January 1976, the
Charles A. Fields Foundation, Ltd. was established
to actively perpetuate the ideals which meant so
much to Charlie. The Foundation's philosophy is
expressed as follows:

> The Officers and Directors of the Fields Foundation,
> Ltd. believe that medical facilities can be more help-
> ful in communities when the public has been edu-
> cated regarding the maintenance of good health.
> They believe that such education can significantly
> reduce the need for acute or crisis medical care.

The Charles A. Fields Foundation, Ltd. hopes to
perpetuate the ideals of an outstanding physician
for the betterment of women's health, and its officers
are proud to have been associated with the production of this book. There is still much that is unknown
or misunderstood about contraceptive methods in
general and about the intrauterine device in par-

ticular. The Foundation hopes that the information presented in this volume will provide health professionals with a better understanding of the medical complications associated with a contraceptive method which has been used by millions of women internationally for two decades.

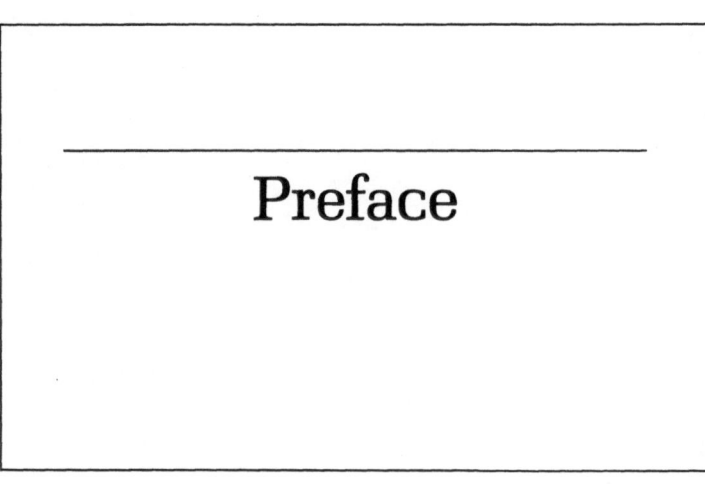

Preface

This collaboration has been a rewarding one for the authors because it has afforded each of us the opportunity to use our individual resources, experiences and perspectives to respond to the need for an objective evaluation of intrauterine devices and their complications. We first identified the need for a review such as this one in 1976 during a series of conversations which focused on the known complications associated with the use of IUDs. A thorough review of the pertinent literature revealed many conflicting results and opinions. This convinced us of the need for an objective overview of the research to date, and ultimately led to our commitment to respond to that need.

Intrauterine Devices and Their Complications is the first comprehensive review of IUDs and their complications to be published and is the result of our evaluation, analysis and synthesis of the reported literature. We think it will provide the reader with a useful overview of significant information which, until now, has not been available in a single document.

We have made a conscious effort to recognize the differences among reported studies and to identify their methodologic limitations so that we might present an accurate and objective appraisal of the complications related to IUD use. Along with our own interpretations, evaluations and assessments, we have provided the reader with summaries of pertinent data from numerous published studies. Most of these summaries have been set off from the text to enhance readability and to identify them for purposes of rapid reference.

It is our hope that this book will reach a wide audience of interested readers and will provide useful information not only for the physician, but also for all individuals interested or involved in any aspect of contraception and reproductive health.

We have tried to be complete as well as concise and have presented all the essential data as succinctly as possible. We hope that the information presented in this book will enhance the reader's ability to assess the value of the IUD and its place in clinical practice, and to evaluate the results of past, present and future research in this field.

We wish to express our deep appreciation to our wives, children, friends and colleagues who have encouraged us and have participated in the preparation of various drafts of the manuscript.

Special acknowledgments for support go to the Charles A. Fields Foundation, the Departments of Obstetrics and Gynecology of Northwestern University and the University of North Carolina at Chapel Hill, the Illinois Family Planning Council and Planned Parenthood of Chicago, Medical Research Consultants, the Menstruation and Reproduction History Research Program and the Center for Reproductive Health.

David A. Edelman
Gary S. Berger
Louis G. Keith

Ocean Isle, North Carolina
May 1979

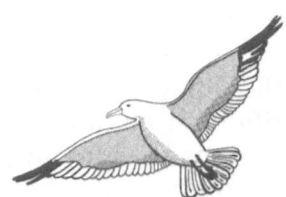

Intrauterine Devices
and Their Complications

Chapter 1

Development, mechanisms of action and evaluation of IUD performance

Early History

The intrauterine device (IUD) is often referred to as a modern medical contraceptive although its origin may be rooted in antiquity. A commonly quoted, but unconfirmed, story dating back to ancient times explains how desert travelers placed small stones in the uteri of their camels to prevent pregnancy during long caravan journeys. The specific observation that intrauterine foreign bodies have an antifertility effect has been credited to Hippocrates.

For centuries, pessaries (Fig. 1.1) with intravaginal stems of wood or bone were inserted through the cervical canal to provide support for internal organs. It was not until the end of the nineteenth century that contraceptive use of stem pessaries was mentioned specifically (7).

In 1909, Richter (34) described an entirely intrauterine contraceptive device which consisted of a loop of silkworm gut (Fig. 1.1). Twenty years later, Grafenberg (10) (Germany) reported experience with over 2,000 women using a ring device made of silver wire wound around a silkworm gut ring (Fig. 1.2). Subsequently, Ota (31) (Japan) further modified the intrauterine ring by replacing the silver wire with gold-plated silver, gold and various plastics (Fig. 1.2). Ota was the first to introduce a type of device which was the forerunner of IUDs as they are known today.

3

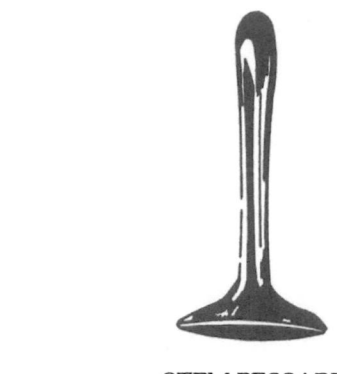

STEM PESSARY

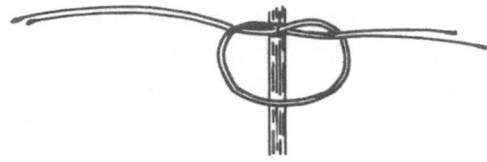

SILKWORM GUT (Richter) IUD

Fig. 1.1: Pessary with intravaginal stem and a silkworm gut (Richter) IUD.

Most gynecologists in both Germany and Japan were opposed to the use of intrauterine rings during the period when Grafenberg and Ota were conducting research. Opposition was based on strong philosophical and cultural objections to the insertion of any foreign body into the uterus, as well as on scientific grounds which suggested that such practices had been associated with pelvic inflammatory disease (PID) in some women. The possibility that PID may have been more common among IUD users than it was among nonusers was not clearly established. Even though Grafenberg and Ota reported a high degree of contraceptive effectiveness for their IUDs, the use of IUDs fell into disrepute.

Widespread interest in the use of IUDs was renewed in 1959 as a result of two reports which marked the beginning of the "modern" era of intra-

uterine contraception. Oppenheimer (30) (Israel) reviewed his 28-year experience with over 1,000
Grafenberg-type ring insertions in 329 women;
Ishihama (19) (Japan) described 973 of his own Ota
ring insertions and reviewed 18,594 insertions by
other physicians. Both investigators reported low
pregnancy rates and the absence of serious side effects or complications.

Recent Developments

IUD development progressed rapidly following the
reports of Oppenheimer and Ishihama. In 1960,
Margulies (USA) developed a spiral-shaped device,
the Gynecoil (Fig. 1.3). For a number of reasons, this
device represented a departure from the previously
accepted design concepts. First, the Gynecoil, or

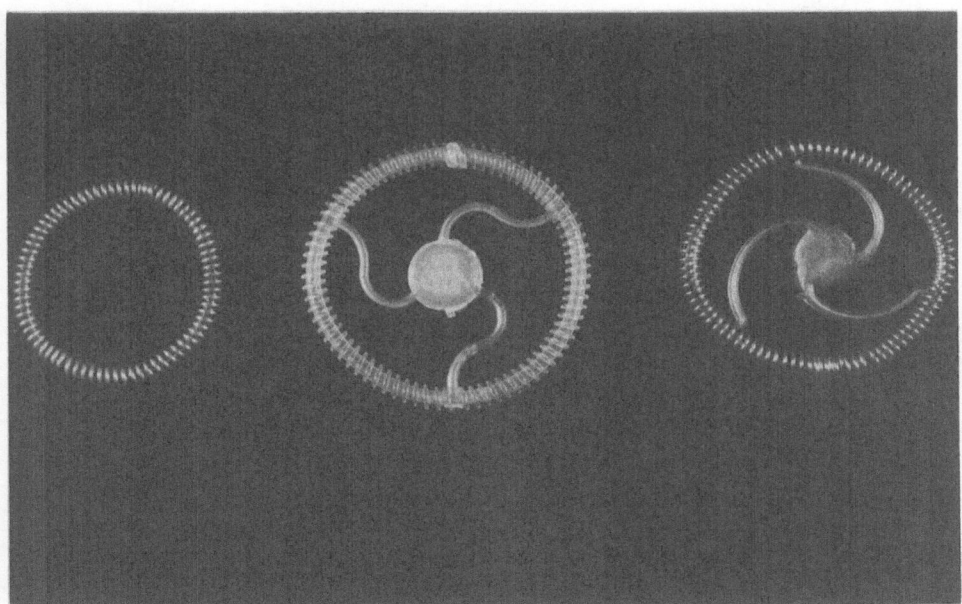

Fig. 1.2: The Gräfenberg Ring and two variations of the Ota
Ring.

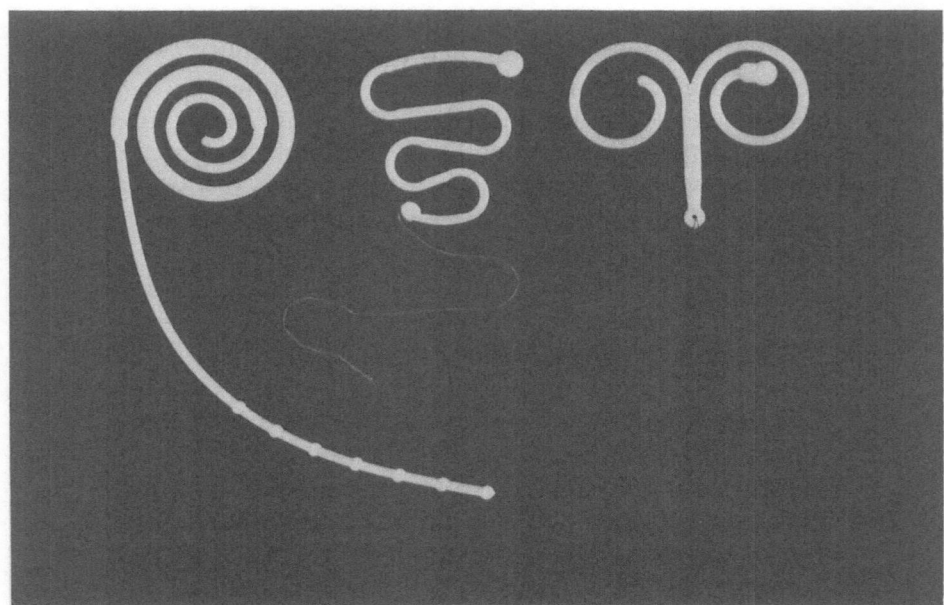

Fig. 1.3: The Margulies Spiral, the Lippes Loop and the Saf-T-Coil.

Margulies spiral, was an "open" device. Since it did not consist of a closed loop or circle, it avoided a design feature which had been associated with severe complications should the device perforate the uterus (herniation and strangulation of a loop of bowel and intra-peritoneal location of the IUD). Second, the stem of the Margulies spiral extended through the cervical canal which facilitated removal of the device. Third, the spiral was made of polyethylene, a plastic polymer which subsequently became the standard for IUD fabrication. Fourth, Margulies incorporated small amounts of barium sulfate into the IUD which made it radiopaque and permitted radiographic identification. Finally, insertion of the device was facilitated by placing the spiral into a narrow plastic tube or carrier which straightened the coil and allowed it to be inserted through the cervical os with minimal dilation. The IUD was then extruded from the carrier and positioned in the uterine cavity where it resumed its original coiled shape.

During the period when Margulies developed his spiral device, Lippes (USA) developed and tested the IUD which bears his name (Fig. 1.3). Of the numerous IUDs that have been developed and tested (Table 1.1), the Lippes Loop has been the most widely used. This IUD is now the standard against which most newer devices are evaluated. Like the Margulies spiral, the Lippes Loop is an "open" device made of polyethylene. The Lippes Loop also contains small amounts of barium sulfate and is inserted into the uterine cavity by extruding it through a narrow plastic tube. The Lippes Loop was the first IUD to use marker strings which extended from the tail of the device through the cervical canal and into the vagina. The purpose of the strings was to facilitate localization and removal of the IUD.

In 1967, Zipper (50) (Chile) made the next sig-

Table 1.1 IUDs that have been evaluated.

Ahmed	Hall-Stone Ring	Quadracoil
Ammeo IUD	Heart	Ragab Ring
Anchor	Hulka	Robinson
Antigon	Icon	Russian Cross
Beospir	Intrauterine Pleated Membrane	Saf-T-Coil
Birnberg Bow	K. S. Wing	Shamrock
Butterfly	Latex Leaf	Silent Protector
China Ring	Lem	Soonawalla Y
Coralle	Lippes Loop	Spira Ring
Cuivre	Louvered Device	Spiran W
Cu-T	M	Spring Coil
Cu-7 (Gravigard)	Marko	Szontagh
Dana	Majzlin Spring	TR-10
Dalkon Shield	Margulies Spiral (Gynecoil)	U-Coil
DIU Pharmatex	Massouras Duck's Foot	Winata
FD-1	Monterrey	Ypsilon
Flower of Canton	Multiload	Yusei Ring
Fluid Filled Tecna	Omega	Zazil Delta A
Ghorbani	Ota Ring	Zipper Ring
Gräfenberg Ring	Progestasert	

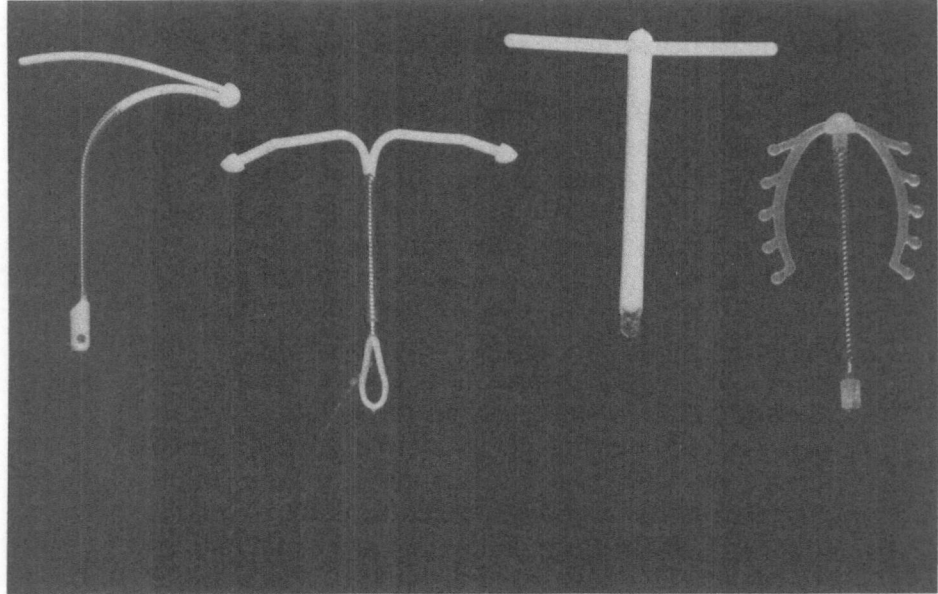

Fig. 1.4: The Cu-7, the Cu-T, the Progestasert and the Multiload.

nificant contribution to the development of the modern IUD. He reported that the placement of a small length of copper wire into one horn of the rabbit uterus greatly reduced the number of implantation sites compared to the contralateral horn into which no copper wire had been placed. Subsequent studies conducted by Zipper and associates (49) demonstrated that a T-shaped device with small amounts of copper wire wrapped around the stem was more effective in reducing the pregnancy rate than was the same device without copper (Fig. 1.4).

   Zipper's discovery marked the beginning of a new generation of IUD development during which antifertility agents (metals, hormones, drugs) were added to the so-called "inert" devices. Further progress in the development of medicated IUDs followed the observations that steroids could permeate dimethylpolysiloxane elastomer (Silastic® Dow-

Corning, Midland, MI) membranes (9,22), and that
the progestin, melengestrol acetate, was shown
histologically to have a progestational effect on uteri
in animal experimentation (8). In 1970, Scommegna
and co-workers (39) reported that the response of the
human endometrium to progesterone released slowly *in utero* from Silastic tubes attached to the upper
arms of Lippes Loops was histologically similar to
that seen after the systemic administration of progestogens. Pandya and Scommegna (32) studied 109
women using progesterone-containing Lippes Loops
which released progesterone at a rate of 300 μg per
day. No pregnancies were reported during 755
woman-months of use. One third of the study subjects noted a decrease in the amount of monthly
bleeding, an effect which was attributed to the local
suppressive effect of progesterone on the endometrium. For the first time, it appeared that the progesterone-releasing modification of IUDs might alleviate
one of the most frequently occurring and undesirable side effects of IUDs, excessive and/or irregular
uterine bleeding.

The progesterone delivery system developed by
Scommegna and associates permitted a rapidly de-
clining rate of hormone release in vivo over time.
This problem was solved by the development of the
Progestasert IUD (Fig. 1.4) which incorporated a
rate-controlling ethylene vinyl acetate copolymer
membrane added to the vertical stem of a T-shaped
device. Tillson and co-workers (45) demonstrated
that the in vivo daily release rate of progesterone
from the Progestasert was stable over a one-year
period and did not differ significantly from the in
vitro release rate of 65 μg per day. Although an
increase in the release rate of progesterone above 65
μg per day would have resulted in an even lower
pregnancy rate (Fig. 1.5), this beneficial effect would
have been negated by a shorter period of time during
which the hormone could be released and would

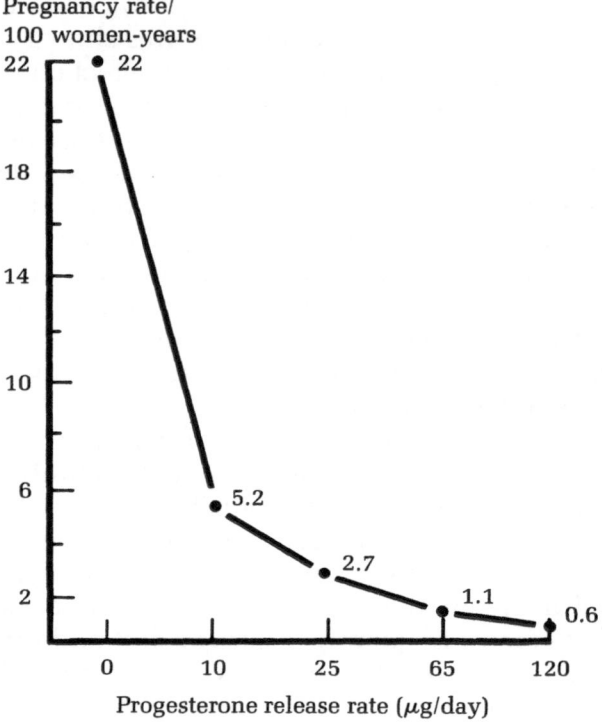

Fig. 1.5: Pregnancy rate associated with rate of progesterone released per day from the Progestasert.

have required that the device be replaced more often than once a year. For this reason, the progesterone release rate of 65 μg per day was selected as the most useful in the clinical setting.

In addition to the Lippes Loop, Saf-T-Coil (Fig. 1.3), Copper-7 (Fig. 1.4), and Progestasert IUDs which are commercially available in the United States today, two other IUDs, the Copper-T and the Multiload, are used extensively in other countries. The Multiload, designed in Holland by Van Os (46), has a polyethylene skeleton with a vertical arm which is wound with copper wire and is appended at the top with two pliable barbed wings (Fig. 1.4).

This design modification was made to increase resistance to expulsion while maintaining the ease of
insertion previously associated with the T-shaped
copper-bearing IUDs.

Mechanisms of Action

General

The mechanisms of action of IUDs have been studied
extensively in many animal species, but the precise
means by which the IUD acts in the human is not
known. Logically, there are four biological events
which may be vulnerable to the action of IUDs:
(1) inhibition or interference with ovulation, (2) interference with fertilization, (3) interference with
blastocyst implantation and (4) early abortion (destruction) of the implanted blastocyst. In addition, it
is possible that the presence of an IUD may influence
coital activity which in turn may affect fertility. This
is of particular importance in certain cultures and
levels of society where intercourse is forbidden any
time a woman has uterine bleeding, regardless of
whether or not it is induced by an IUD. There is no
evidence to suggest that any type of IUD (nonmedicated, copper-bearing or progesterone-releasing)
acts by inhibiting ovulation. However, there is conflicting evidence regarding the possible interference
of IUDs with fertilization, nidation and subsequent
growth of the blastocyst.

Although there are a variety of IUD-related antifertility effects in different animal species, the single
factor common to all species is the IUD's ability to
evoke a local inflammatory response in the endometrium. In a recent review (21), it was suggested that
macrophages and polymorphonuclear leukocytes
which surround the IUD may promote an accumula-
tion of embryotoxic materials within the uteri of

rodents. Studies in humans, however, have not supported such activity as a primary mechanism of action. On the other hand, it has been observed among primates that macrophages phagocytize spermatozoa.

Recent biochemical studies suggest that IUDs alter the response of the human endometrium to endogenous ovarian hormones which in turn may interfere with nidation of the blastocyst. If fertilization does occur, and the developing blastocyst is prevented from implanting successfully in the uterus, then one might find evidence to confirm the presence of very early pregnancy in IUD users. Some investigators (4,24) have reported elevated plasma human chorionic gonadotropin (HCG) levels in some IUD users (12−19%) during the luteal phase of their menstrual cycles suggesting that these women may have been pregnant and then aborted. Other investigators have been unable to confirm these findings (2,23). Therefore, the questions regarding the effects of the IUD on nidation of the blastocyst remain unresolved.

Systemic Immune Response

A number of investigators have suggested that the action of IUDs may be initiated through changes in the immune response system which prevent the unusual immune tolerance of the mother to the developing embryo. Evidence in support of an altered immune response are the increased levels of serum immunoglobulins A, G and M following the insertion of a variety of IUDs (12,18,28).

Prostaglandins

The prostaglandins have been hypothesized to take part in the mechanisms of action of IUDs by their ability to increase uterine activity and interfere either with implantation or with the growth of the implanted blastocyst.

Chaudhuri (5) postulated that the IUD may provoke prostaglandin release from the endometrium as a result of trauma. Subsequently, Myatt and co-workers (29) found that macrophages adherent to a variety of IUDs removed for "routine" reasons were a likely source of prostaglandin activity (primarily PGF).

Other investigators (11,17), however, have not found increased levels of PGF or its metabolites among IUD users. Hillier and Kasonde (17) did find a significant increase in endometrial PGE concentrations in 11 of 14 women examined one to five months after IUD insertion compared to concentrations found before insertion. A variety of IUDs were used in the study, but increased PGE levels did not appear to be associated with any particular IUD.

The equivocal nature of these findings is underscored when one considers that other factors, such as the phase of the menstrual cycle, may be more closely associated with prostaglandin activity than is the presence or absence of an IUD.

Medicated IUDs

While small IUDs may be better tolerated by women than larger ones, they are associated with higher pregnancy rates (Table 1.2). The addition of antifertility agents to IUDs permits the use of small IUDs without compromising their effectiveness. In addition to any effect derived from the presence of the plastic carrier *in utero*, the medicated IUDs have other qualities which improve their contraceptive effectiveness. This is true for both copper-bearing and progesterone-releasing IUDs. The T-IUD without copper and the placebo Progestasert both have

Table 1.2 Relationship between IUD surface area and
pregnancy rates

IUD	Surface Area (mm²)	Pregnancy Rate*
Small Birnberg Bow	390	17.0
Lippes Loop A	527	11.7
Large Birnberg Bow	816	8.6
Lippes Loop D	960	4.9
Small Margulies Spiral	960	5.4
Large Margulies Spiral	1,200	2.9

* Two-year gross life table rates per 100 women.
SOURCE: Adapted from Tietze and Lewit (43).

higher failure rates than their medicated counter-
parts. Furthermore, the effectiveness of these IUDs
has been correlated with the daily release rate of the
bioactive drug, in the case of Progestasert, and with
the total copper surface area of the copper-bearing
IUD (Figs. 1.5 and 1.6).

Copper-bearing IUDs The copper portion of a copper-bearing IUD has a significant contraceptive effect
which is quite apart from any effect of the inert
carrier. This was demonstrated by Zipper and co-
workers (48) in a study of 32 women, each of whom
had a copper wire inserted which was 32 cm in
length and 0.2 mm in diameter with a surface area
of 200 mm² when wound around a narrow polyethylene thread (0.1 mm in diameter, 2.5 cm in
length). During 348 woman-months of exposure, the
pregnancy rate was 3.4 per 100 woman-years of use.
This rate was only slightly higher than the pregnancy rate associated with the Cu-T-200.
    The failure rate associated with some copper-
bearing IUDs (Cu-T) can be reduced by adding up to
200 mm² of exposed copper surface area (Fig. 1.6).
Increasing the copper surface area beyond 200 mm²
has no apparent effect on pregnancy rates. The daily
copper release rate apparently is not the critical fac-

tor as it declines from 60 μg per day during the initial months of use to less than 10 μg per day during the second and third years of use (42) when the failure rate is lower than in the initial months (51).

Studies on the contraceptive mechanisms of action of copper are inconclusive.

Hefnawi and co-workers (16) reported that the cervical mucus of Copper T users showed less ferning and spinnbarkeit, had greater turbidity and was more hostile to sperm penetration and motility than the cervical mucus of either Lippes Loop users or non-users of IUDs. These observations, however, have not been confirmed by others (6,36). Hagenfeldt (14) concluded that sperm motility might be inhibited during the first few months following IUD insertion when

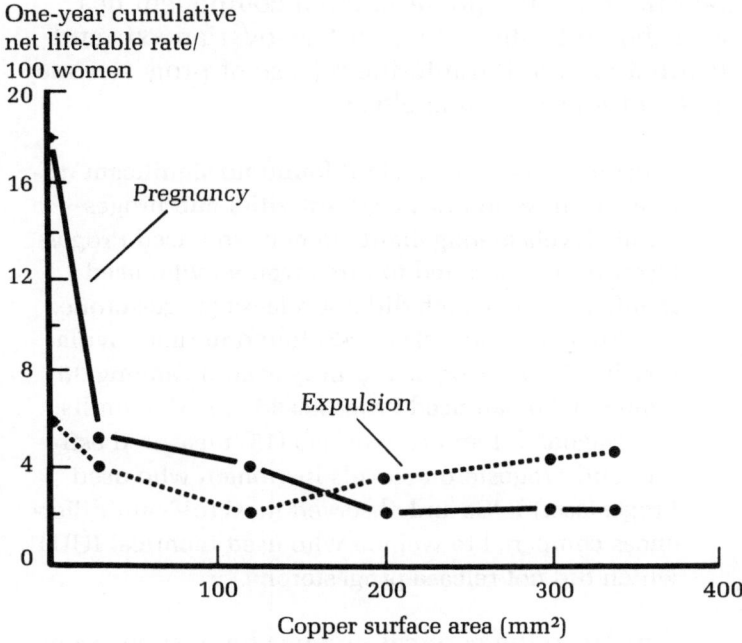

Fig. 1.6: Pregnancy and expulsion rates associated with the amount of exposed copper surface area on the Cu-T.

the copper concentration in the uterine fluids and cervical mucus was highest. In a review of the literature, Hagenfeldt found no evidence for an effect of copper on ovulation or ovarian function.

Rather than affecting sperm motility, it seems more likely that copper changes the uterine milieu causing it to inhibit implantation, since a number of metabolic changes occur in the endometrium at midcycle when implantation might normally be expected to take place. According to Hagenfeldt (14), the local inflammatory reaction seen in association with copper-bearing IUDs does not in itself appear sufficient to explain their greater efficacy compared to that of the inert carriers.

Progesterone-releasing IUDs Unlike oral contraceptives in which the progestational component has been shown to affect the pituitary-ovarian axis and its function, the intrauterine release of progesterone apparently has no such effect.

> Tillson and co-workers (45) found no significant differences in serum LH, FSH, estradiol and progesterone levels among eight women who used Progestasert IUDs compared to three women who used identical IUDs which did not release progesterone.
> Wan and co-workers (47) found normal, ovulatory levels of estrogen and progesterone among 38 women who had used Progestaserts for 12 months.
> Hagenfeldt and co-workers (15) measured estradiol and progesterone levels in women who used Progestasert IUDs and observed no significant differences compared to women who used identical IUDs which did not release progesterone.

Similar to the cervical mucus changes observed in women using copper-bearing IUDs, the progesterone-releasing IUDs also appear to affect cervical mucus so that sperm penetration may be impaired (26). In addition, there is evidence that endometrial secretions impair normal sperm physiology in the presence of a progesterone-releasing IUD (35).

The key to the effectiveness of the progesterone-releasing IUD probably lies in its local hormonal action on the endometrium, which impairs implantation of the blastocyst. The major histologic effects associated with IUDs which release progesterone include decidual reaction, glandular atrophy and an inflammatory response. These findings become more frequent as the dose of progesterone is increased, as well as with the increasing duration of IUD use (3,15,27).

The suppression of endometrial proliferation has been demonstrated by a reduction in nuclear DNA content in endometrial epithelial cells (20). Among the observed biochemical changes are a reduction in alkaline phosphatase and beta glucoronidase, an increase in acid phosphatase and a variable effect on lactic dehydrogenase activity, depending on the phase of the menstrual cycle (13). An additional effect, also observed in association with copper-bearing IUDs, is a decrease in endometrial zinc levels during the luteal phase of the cycle.

Although most information suggests that the primary mechanism of action of the progesterone-releasing IUD is to inhibit implantation of the blastocyst, there is also some evidence which suggests that changes occur in the uterine contractility patterns which might disrupt the developing embryo. Ruiz-Velasco and co-workers (37) found that uterine contractions increased in intensity but decreased in frequency under the influence of the Progestasert. Whether changes in uterine contractility are important to the contraceptive mechanisms of the Progestasert or any other IUD has not yet been determined.

Evaluation of IUD Performance

A major difficulty encountered in any attempt to
compare a variety of reported IUD complication rates
centers around the fact that various investigators use
different methods of reporting their data. In the years
prior to the adaptation of the life table method of
analysis for the evaluation of contraceptive effectiveness, the effectiveness of IUDs often was reported as
a percentage of the numbers of women using the
IUD or in terms of the events per 100 woman-years of
IUD use. The latter statistic, the Pearl Index, is computed as:

$$\frac{\text{Number of Events}}{\text{Total Woman-Months of IUD Use}} \times 1{,}200$$

The major disadvantage of the Pearl Index is that it
does not take into account *when* events occur. For
events which occur during the follow-up period,
neither of these methods is satisfactory, since they
do not take into account the duration of follow-up
and the number or proportion of women for whom
follow-up data are available. Following their IUD insertion, women discontinue use at different times
and for different reasons. The number of women
using any IUD changes continually and procedures
for evaluating IUD performance should take all of
these factors into account.

The presently accepted method of evaluating
IUD performance is the life table method. This approach can be used to compute the probability of
occurrence of IUD-related events as a function of
time from IUD insertion. The two basic assumptions
which underlie use of the life table method are:
(1) the risks of terminating IUD use for any reason
may depend on the length of time since IUD insertion, but are the same for all women at any time interval from IUD insertion; and (2) women who are
lost to follow-up have essentially the same IUD experience as women who are not lost to follow-up.

The basic data required for the computation of life table rates include: (1) the duration of IUD use from the insertion for each continuing IUD user, (2) the duration of IUD use from insertion to discontinuation for all women who have withdrawn from observation and (3) the reasons for withdrawal, (e.g., pregnancy, expulsion, removal, lost from further observation). Time is usually measured in months, but any unit of time may be used. The data are then used to calculate net or gross life table rates for each type of IUD event. These rates are computed for each unit or time and as a cumulative rate over time.

The difference between net and gross life table rates is illustrated in terms of pregnancy rates. The net pregnancy rate is calculated on the basis that women may leave the study for reasons other than pregnancy, such as expulsion or removal, before they have had a chance to become pregnant. On the other hand, the gross pregnancy rate provides an estimate of the pregnancy rate as if pregnancy were the *only* reason for withdrawal from observation. Both net and gross rates give event probabilities per woman, or rates per 100 women, and can be computed for any duration of IUD use. The net rates for all possible termination reasons add up exactly to the total termination rate for all reasons combined. Net rates are used to report the experience of a group of women using one type of IUD. Gross rates should be used for the comparison of specific events for two or more IUDs or groups of women. Detailed procedures for the computation of net and gross life table rates have been published by Potter (33) and by Tietze and Lewit (44).

Table 1.3 shows the one-year net cumulative rates of the pregnancy, expulsion and medical removal rates for IUDs which are commercially available in the United States (Lippes Loop, sizes A, B, C, D; Saf-T-Coil, sizes 25S, 32S, 33S; Cu-7-200—Gravigard; Progestasert). These rates are reprinted from product information supplied by the manu-

Table 1.3 *One-year net cumulative life table rates per 100 women for IUDs commercially available in the United States.*

	Number of Insertions	Pregnancy	Expulsion	Medical Removal
Lippes Loop*				
Size A	1,015	5.3	23.9	12.2
B	1,305	3.4	18.9	15.1
C	3,489	3.0	19.1	14.3
D	7,553	2.7	12.7	15.2
Saf-T-Coil†				
(All Sizes)	NS‡	2.4	18.3	15.6
Cu-7				
(Gravigard§)				
Nulliparas	NS‖	1.6	8.0	13.7
Multiparas	NS	1.9	5.7	10.7
Progestasert#				
Nulliparas	} 7,614	2.6	7.4	15.1
Multiparas		1.8	3.1	11.2

* Ortho Pharmaceutical Corporation, Raritan, N.J., USA (43)
† Schmidt Laboratories Inc., Little Falls, N.J., USA (38)
‡ Not stated; 4,231 women completed 12 months of use.
§ Searle Laboratories, Chicago, Ill., USA (40)
‖ Not stated; 11,852 women completed 12 months of IUD use.
Alza Pharmaceuticals, Palo Alto, Calif., USA. (1)

facturers of the IUDs, or from data sources referenced by the manufacturers.

Summary

The two thousand years between the time of Hippocrates and the beginning of the twentieth century evidenced little progress in the area of intrauterine contraception. Then, in the first half of the 1900s, pioneers such as Ota and Gräfenberg demonstrated the effectiveness of IUDs. Their work eventually led to the modification and widespread use of IUDs in the 1960s and 1970s. Following the favorable reports

of Ishihama (19) and Oppenheimer (30) in 1959 on
the long-term use of IUDs, numerous IUDs were developed and evaluated, including copper-bearing
and progesterone-releasing IUDs. Of the numerous
IUDs developed during the twentieth century only
four are commercially available today in the United
States: Lippes Loop, Saf-T-Coil, Cu-7 and Progestasert.

During the past two decades, numerous investigators have attempted to explain the mechanisms of
contraceptive action of IUDs. The known mechanisms vary widely and are dependent upon the
species of animal studied and on the specific IUD
used. The exact mechanism of action in humans remains to be elucidated. The consensus of opinion,
however, is that the existence of a local inflammatory reaction appears to play an important role for
all IUDs, with additional modes of action in effect for
the medicated IUDs.

Reported studies on IUD effectiveness and other
IUD-related events have varied according to the eval-
uative methods utilized. The currently preferred
method used to analyze and report IUD performance
data is the life-table method. This method provides
estimates of the probabilities of IUD-related events
as a function of time from insertion, whereas the
Pearl Index and other methods do not.

References

1. Alza Pharmaceuticals. *The Progestasert*. Intrauterine
   progesterone contraceptive system release rated 65
   μg/day progesterone for one year. Alza Product Information, Palo Alto, California, 1977.

2. Aubert, J. M.; Boria, M. C.; Stone, M. L.; and Reyniak,
   J. V. Assessment of human chorionic gonadotropin
   (hCG) levels during luteal phase in women using intrauterine contraception. *Contraception* 16:557, 1977.

3. Aznar, R.; Lozano, M.; and Martinez-Manautou, J. Contraception with progesterone-releasing intrauterine systems. *Ginecol. Obstet. Mex.* 37:69, 1975.

4. Beling, C. G.; Cederqvist, L. L.; and Fuchs, F. Demonstration of gonadotropin during the second half of the cycle in women using intrauterine contraception. *Am. J. Obstet. Gynecol.* 125:855, 1976.

5. Chaudhuri, G. Intrauterine device: possible role of prostaglandins. *Lancet* 2:480, 1971.

6. Duanter, B.; Chantler, E. N.; and Elstein, M. The scanning electronmicroscopy of human cervical mucus in the non-pregnant and pregnant states. *Br. J. Obstet. Gynaecol.* 3:738, 1976.

7. Davis, H. J. *Intrauterine devices for contraception. The IUD.* Baltimore: Williams and Wilkins Company, 1971.

8. Doyle, L. L., and Clewe, T. H. Preliminary studies on the effect of hormone-releasing intrauterine devices. *Am. J. Obstet. Gynecol.* 101:564, 1968.

9. Dziuk, P. J., and Cook, B. Passage of steroids through silicone rubber. *Endocrinology* 78:208, 1966.

10. Grafenberg, E. Die intrauterine method der konzeption-suerhutung. In *Intrauterine contraceptive rings: history and statistical appraisal. III congress World League for Sexual Reform.* International Congress Series, No. 54. Amsterdam: Excerpta Medical, 1929.

11. Green, K., and Hagenfeldt, K. Prostaglandins in the human endometrium. Gas chromatographic-mass spectrometric quantitation before and after IUD insertion. *Am. J. Obstet. Gynecol.* 122:611, 1975.

12. Gump, D. W.; Mead, P. B.; Horton, E. L.; Lamborn, K. R.; and Forsyth, B. R. Intrauterine contraceptive device and increased serum immunoglobulin levels. *Obstet. Gynecol.* 41:259, 1975.

13. Hagenfeldt, K. Intrauterine contraception with the Copper-T device. 1. Effect on trace elements in the endometrium, cervical mucus and plasma. *Contraception* 6:37, 1972.

14. Hagenfeldt, K. The modes of action of medicated intrauterine devices. *J. Reprod. Fertil.*, (Suppl) 25:117, 1976.

15. Hagenfeldt, K.; Landgren, B-M; Edstrom, K.; and Johannisson, E. Biochemical and morphological changes in the human endometrium induced by the Progestasert device. *Contraception* 16:183, 1977.

16. Hefnawi, F.; Kandil, O.; Askalani, H.; and Serour, G. Influence of the copper IUD and the Lippes Loop on sperm migration in the human cervical mucus. *Contraception* 11:541, 1975.

17. Hillier, K., and Kasonde, J. M. Prostaglandin E and F concentrations in human endometrium after insertion of intrauterine contraceptive device. *Lancet* I:15, 1976.

18. Holub, W. R.; Reyner, F. C.; and Forman, G. H. Increased levels of serum immunoglobulins and G and M in women using intrauterine contraceptive devices. *Am. J. Obstet. Gynecol.* 110:362, 1971.

19. Ishihama, A. Clinical studies on intrauterine rings. Especially the present state of contraception in Japan and the experiences in the use of intrauterine rings. *Yokahama. Med. Bull.* 10:89, 1959.

20. Johannisson, F.; Landgren, B-M; and Hagenfeldt, K. The effect of intrauterine progesterone on the DNA-content in isolated human endometrial cells. *Acta. Cytol.* 21:441, 1977.

21. Joshi, S. G. Local effects of pharmacologically inert IUDs in rats, baboons, and humans. In *Analysis of intrauterine contraception*, eds. F. Hefnawi, and S. J. Segal. New York: American Elsevier Publishing Co., 1975.

22. Kincl, F. A.; Benagiano, G.; and Angee, I. Sustained release hormonal preparations. I. Diffusion of various steroids through polymer membranes. *Steroids* 11:673, 1968.

23. Klein, T. A., and Mishell, D. E. Absence of circulating chorionic gonadotropin in wearers of intrauterine contraceptive devices. *Am. J. Obstet. Gynecol.* 129:626, 1977.

24. Landesman, R.; Coutinho, E. M.; and Saxena, B. B. Detection of human chorionic gonadotropin in blood of regularly bleeding women using copper intrauterine devices. *Fertil. Steril.* 27:1062, 1976.

25. Martinez-Manautou, J. Contraception by intrauterine release of progesterone. Clinical studies. *J. Steroid Biochem.* 6:889, 1975.

26. Martinez-Manautou, J.; Aznar, R.; Maqueo, M.; and Pharriss, B. B. Uterine Therapeutic system for long-term contraception: II. Clinical correlates. *Fertil. Steril.* 25:922, 1974.

27. Martinez-Manautou, J.; Correu-Azcona, S., and Aznar-Ramos, R. Experience in Mexico with the intrauterine hormone contraceptive system (three years of research). *Ginec. Obstet. Mex.* 40:61, 1976.

28. Mountrose, U. E.; Whitehouse, W. L.; and Slater, L. Serum immunoglobulins and C-reactive protein in patients using intrauterine contraceptive devices. *Br. J. Obstet. Gynaecol.* 82:992, 1975.

29. Myatt, L.; Bray, M. A.; Gordon, D.; and Morley, J. Macrophages on intrauterine contraceptive devices produce prostaglandins. *Nature* 257:227, 1975.

30. Oppenheimer, W. Prevention of pregnancy by the Grafenberg Ring method: a re-evaluation after 28 years' experience. *Am. J. Obstet. Gynecol.* 78:446, 1959.

31. Ota, T. A study on birth control with an intrauterine instrument. *Jap. J. Obstet. Gynecol.* 17:210, 1934.

32. Pandya, G. N., and Scommegna, A. Intrauterine progesterone-releasing devices: a clinical trial. *Adv. Plann. Parent.* VII, 103, 1971.

33. Potter, R. G. Use-effectiveness of intrauterine contraception as a problem in competing risks. In *Family planning in Taiwan*, eds. R. Freedman, and J. Takeshita, New Jersey: Princeton University Press, 1969.

34. Richter, R. Ein mittel zus verhutung der konzeption. *Deutsche Medizinische Wochenschrift* 35:1525, 1909.

35. Rosado, A.; Hicks, J. J.; Aznar, R.; and Mercado, E. Intrauterine contraception with the progesterone-T device. *Contraception* 9:39, 1974.

36. Rush, F., and Elstein, M. The effect of incubating a copper releasing intrauterine device on sperm penetration and spinnbarkeit of cervical mucus. *J. Obstet. Gynaecol. Brit. Comnwlth.* 81:483, 1974.

37. Ruiz-Velasco, V.; Martinez-Manautou, J.; Amuriio, S. I.; Salinas, G. R.; Topete, M. M.; and Conde de Vargas, B. I. The active intrauterine system in dysfunctional uterine bleeding. Its effect on the myometrium, endometrium, and vaginal epithelium. *J. Brazil. Ginecol.* 78:417, 1974.

38. Schmidt Laboratories. Saf-T-Coil Product Information, Little Falls, N.J.

39. Scommegna, A.; Pandya, G. N.; Christ, M.; Lee, A. W.; and Cohen, M. R. Intrauterine administration of progesterone by a slow releasing device. *Fertil. Steril.* 21:201, 1970.

40. Searle Laboratories. Cu-7 brand of intrauterine copper contraceptive. Searle Laboratories Product Information, Chicago, Illinois, 1977.

41. Shulman, G.; Polakow, E. S.; and Bauer, H. D. Serum immunoglobulin levels in women using intrauterine contraceptive devices. *J. Obstet. Gynaecol. Br. Comnwlth.* 81:155, 1974.

42. Stewart, W. C.; O'Brien, F. B.; Nissen, C.; and Deysach, L. Multiclinic evaluation of Gravigard (Cu-7) intrauterine contraception. In *Analysis of intrauterine contraception*, eds. F. Hefnawi and S. J. Segal. New York: American Elsevier Publishing Co., 1975.

43. Tietze, C., and Lewit, S. Evaluation of intrauterine devices: ninth progress report of the Cooperative Statistical Program. *Stud. Fam. Plann.* No. 59, July 1970.

44. Tietze, C., and Lewit, S. Recommended procedures for the statistical evaluation of intrauterine contraception. *Stud. Fam. Plann.* 4(2):35, 1973.

45. Tillson, S. A.; Marian, M.; Hudson, R.; Wong, P.; Pharriss, B.; Aznar, R.; and Martinez-Manautou, J. The effect of intrauterine progesterone on the hypothalmic-hypophyseal-ovarian axis in humans. *Contraception* 11:179, 1975.

46. Van Os, W. A. A.; Rhemsey, P. E. R.; Bomert, L.; and Aartsen, E. J. Experience with a combined multiload contraceptive intrauterine device. Paper presented at 8th World Congress on Fertility and Sterility, November 3–9, 1974, Buenos Aires, Argentina.

47. Wan, L. S.; Hsu, Y-C.; Ganguly, M.; and Bigelow, B. Effects of Progestasert on the menstrual pattern, ovarian steroids and endometrium. *Contraception* 16:417, 1977.

48. Zipper, J.; Edelman, D. A.; and Goldsmith, A. An overview of IUD research and implications for the future. *Int. J. Gynaecol. Obstet.* 15:73, 1977.

49. Zipper, J.; Medel, M.; Pastene, L.; and Rivera, M. Factors that limit the efficiency of copper-carrying IUDs.

In *Intrauterine devices: development, evaluation and program implementation*, eds. R. G. Wheeler, G. W. Duncan, and J. J. Speidel. New York: Academic Press, 1974.

50. Zipper, J.; Medel, M.; and Prager, R. Suppression of fertility by intrauterine copper and zinc in rabbits. *Am. J. Obstet. Gynecol.* 105:529, 1969.

51. Zipper, J.; Medel, M.; Osorio, A.; Goldsmith, A.; and Edelman, D. A. Long-term use effectiveness of the Cu-7-200 IUD. *Int. J. Gynaecol. Obstet.* 14:142, 1976.

Chapter 2

IUD
insertion

Introduction

IUD complications may occur at the time of insertion and/or at some later time. Complications which affect the ease and safety of IUD insertion may be related to patient selection, choice of IUD, timing of the insertion or inadequate insertion technique.

Patient Selection

Not every woman is a candidate for successful intra-uterine contraception. The contraindications to IUD use include:

1. known or suspected pregnancy
2. active pelvic inflammatory disease
3. cancer of the cervix or uterus
4. abnormal uterine bleeding
5. uterine fibroids
6. cervical stenosis
7. severe displacement of the uterus
8. structural or anatomic abnormalities such as bicornuate or septate uterus
9. anemia, menorrhagia and severe dysmenorrhea
10. prior pelvic inflammatory disease
11. prior ectopic pregnancy
12. history of valvular heart disease.

At present, there is no uniform agreement as to whether each of the 12 items represents a relative or an absolute contraindication, although most authorities consider any one of the first four items to be an absolute contraindication to IUD use. Each of the remaining items must be evaluated carefully before a clinical decision can be made either to use or not use an IUD.

Known or Suspected Pregnancy

Pregnancy termination is not the inevitable consequence of an IUD insertion that occurs early in the course of a pregnancy. The insertion of an IUD per se does not invariably induce abortion although some clinicians who practiced in the days before legal abortion may have inserted IUDs into pregnant patients to cause bleeding that necessitated a curettage.

The IUD cannot be recommended as an effective or safe abortifacient, but its insertion after unprotected, midcycle coitus may interfere with the implantation of the blastocyst (23).

> Lippes and co-workers (23) inserted Cu-7 IUDs into 97 noncontracepting women one to five days after exposure to the risk of pregnancy at midcycle. No pregnancies occurred within three months of the postcoital insertion, and there were no reported complications.

If the patient is pregnant, the pregnancy should be terminated before the IUD is inserted. Insertion of an IUD immediately after an abortion does not increase the risks of complications.

Active Pelvic Inflammatory Disease

Evidence has accumulated in recent years which indicates an increased risk of acute pelvic inflammatory disease (PID) among IUD users (see Chapter 4). The routine proscription against inserting an IUD during the acute phase of PID is logical, since it is presumed that the introduction of a foreign body into an inflamed uterus might intensify the infectious process. To our knowledge, however, no data have been reported which actually document the sequelae of such activity.

A cervical culture for gonorrhea should be performed routinely prior to or at the time of IUD insertion, as there is always the risk that an IUD may be inserted into a woman with an occult or subclinical genital tract infection. In the event of a positive culture, rapid patient contact and treatment is essential, as are efforts to trace and treat the patient's recent sexual partner(s). An infected patient who is asymptomatic at the time of treatment need not have her IUD removed. In the symptomatic patient, there are insufficient data to assist the clinician in determining whether the infection should be treated with the IUD in situ or after it has been removed.

Cancer of the Cervix or Uterus

There is no evidence to suggest that the IUD plays an etiologic role in the development of uterine or cervical cancer (see Chapter 6). There are good reasons, however, for the generally accepted restriction against the insertion of an IUD into a woman with known or suspected cancer of the uterus or cervix. First, the IUD cannot promote the return to health of an individual who suffers from malignant disease; in fact, it may impede or hinder the initiation of appropriate therapy. Second, the most common symptoms associated with IUD use (irregular bleeding and varying degrees of lower abdominal discomfort) also may occur when pelvic malignancy exists. Thus, the diagnosis of cancer of the cervix or uterus may be overlooked even when symptoms are pro-

tracted because they may be attributed to the IUD. It
is a matter of major concern that the IUD may be
considered the cause of abnormal uterine bleeding
which, in fact, may be attributed to an existing
disease which requires treatment. Undiagnosed
cancer is the most serious, but unlikely, possibility.

It should be noted that dysplastic lesions of the
cervix are not a contraindication to IUD insertion.
There is no evidence to suggest that the insertion of
an IUD will cause dysplasia to progress more rapidly
to carcinoma in situ.

Uterine Fibroids

The presence of intramural or submucosal fibroids
(leiomyoma) may contribute to a general distortion
of the uterine cavity. Insertion may be more difficult,
and proper fundal placement may not be possible. If
an IUD is inserted under such conditions, there is an
increased likelihood of subsequent pregnancy and/
or expulsion. In rare instances, the IUD may become
embedded in the myoma (11). Bimanual palpation of
the uterus cannot provide complete and essential
information; only hysterosalpingography or hysteroscopy can provide the essential evidence required
to determine the extent of endometrial cavity distortion.

Cervical Stenosis

This condition occurs in parous as well as nulliparous women. No IUD should be inserted without first
demonstrating cervical patency. Usually this is ac-
complished when the uterus is sounded for its total
axial length and direction of the cervical canal. The
insertion of an IUD into a patient with a stenotic cervix carries with it the risk of cervical laceration, pro-

duction of a false cervical passage and uterine perforation.

Severe Displacement of the Uterus

IUD insertion should be attempted only with the utmost care in those instances when the uterocervical axis cannot be straightened by traction on the cervix with a tenaculum. Anterior wall perforations at the time of IUD insertion occur more commonly in retroverted uteri, while posterior wall perforations are more common in anteverted uteri (see Chapter 3).

Structural or Anatomic Deformities

Failure to recognize intrauterine anatomic abnormalities may substantially increase the risk of unwanted pregnancy, even if the IUD is inserted. Although it may be physically possible to insert an IUD into each horn of a bicornuate uterus, this cannot be recommended as a standard procedure. Vago and Spira (37) reported a case of pregnancy in one uterine compartment, while the other was protected with an IUD.

Anemia, Menorrhagia and Dysmenorrhea

Anemia and menorrhagia may be worsened after an IUD insertion because of the increased blood loss associated with IUD use. Women with these disorders who desire intrauterine contraception might best be served by the Progestasert IUD since this device is associated with decreased menstrual flow and, in some instances, diminished menstrual discomfort.

Prior Pelvic Inflammatory Disease

The term "chronic PID" represents a variety of clinical conditions, only some of which are associated
with a history of an acute, documented inflammatory
process. There is no way to tell whether or not
chronic PID will become active after an IUD insertion any more than it is possible to predict which
patients with subclinical infections will develop
clinical symptomatology after the IUD insertion. It is
best to avoid the insertion of an IUD into a woman
with prior or chronic PID unless no other contraceptive possibility is acceptable and contraception is
essential.

Prior History of Ectopic Pregnancy

A woman with a prior ectopic pregnancy is at a higher risk of a subsequent ectopic pregnancy (13,32)
than is a woman without such a history. The association between IUD use and ectopic pregnancy (see
Chapter 8) suggests that a woman with a prior history of such pregnancy should avoid using an IUD.
It is thought that IUD insertion might increase the
risk of PID, and in this manner, contribute to an even
greater risk of ectopic pregnancy.

History of Valvular Heart Disease

Insertion of the IUD results in transient bacterial
contamination of the endometrial cavity and occasionally may be associated with severe bacterial pelvic infection. The greatest caution should be exer-
ised in deciding whether or not to insert an IUD in a
woman with a history of bacterial endocarditis or in
a woman with a history of rheumatic fever who has
evidence of valvular damage. In such cases, there

may be a risk of bacteremia and further infectious damage to the cardiac valves. To our knowledge, there are no published series of IUD use among patients with rheumatic heart disease. Therefore, each request for IUD insertion made by a woman with a history of valvular heart disease must be considered on an individual basis.

IUD Selection

A number of investigators recently have shown that the means exist for the rational selection of a specific IUD for individual patients. If such a selection procedure is followed, the incidence of late complications or undesirable events can be lowered. The ability to select the proper IUD for an individual acceptor stems from the knowledge that there are great disparities in the endometrial cavity size (all dimensions) in different uteri which have the same overall length from external os to fundus (14).

> Tejuja and Malkani (36) demonstrated that the frequency of IUD associated bleeding and pain was probably related to the disparity between the size of the uterus and the IUD.
>
> Wheeler and co-workers (38) evaluated certain mechanical properties (size, thickness, surface area, volume, transverse and longitudinal bowing, transverse and longitudinal compression) of various non-medicated IUDs and found these properties to be predictive for pregnancy, expulsion and pain and/or bleeding removal rates.
>
> Hasson and co-workers (14) recorded a significantly higher rate of events (pregnancy, expulsion or removal for medical reasons) when the length of the IUD was two or more centimeters longer or shorter than the length of the endometrial cavity (internal os to fundus).

The obvious implication of the studies of Tejuja and Malkani (36) and Hasson and co-workers (14) is that improved results could be obtained with the available IUDs if an IUD of appropriate size were selected for each woman. While the prescriptive approach to IUD fitting has been mentioned in the literature with considerable frequency, there does not exist sufficient information to provide physicians with a rational set of decision-making rules.

Timing of Insertion

An IUD may be inserted at any time during the menstrual cycle, as well as after abortion or term delivery.

Interval (Nonabortal, Nonpuerperal) Insertion

There are several advantages to the insertion of an IUD during menstruation. First, menstrual insertion avoids the inadvertent disruption of an unrecognized or early pregnancy. Second, the cervical canal is more likely to be dilated, facilitating insertion. Third, bleeding secondary to the insertion is indistinguishable from menstrual blood and thus may alleviate a source of patient anxiety. Finally, the rates of postinsertion complications may be diminished when insertions are performed during menstruation.

Akinla and co-workers (3) studied the effect of the timing of Cu-T insertion in 2,689 women. The rate of removals for all reasons at 12 months was lower (4.8 per 100 women) for women who received insertions on the first three days of their menstrual cycles and increased to a maximum of 12.9 per 100 women for insertions performed after day 21. The 12-month removal rates for pain and bleeding for insertions performed on the first three days and after day 21 of the menstrual cycle were 2.9 and 8.3 per 100 women, respectively. Also of interest was the observation of a higher 12-month expulsion rate (3.2 per 100 women) after midcycle insertions (days 8–14) compared to all other times of insertion (1.1 to 1.9 per 100 women for days 1–7 and days 15 and on). The authors postulated that the higher expulsion rate associated with midcycle insertions might have resulted from expulsion during the insertional cycle due to increased myometrial activity.

In contrast to Akinla's report, a review of 2,390 Dalkon Shield insertions showed no significant differences in the pregnancy, expulsion or medical removal rates for bleeding, pain or other reasons at any time during the first year of use between women who had their IUD inserted during menstruation and those who did not (1).

It is difficult to weigh the significance of the observations made by Akinla and co-workers since their conclusions are based on 12-month event rates rather than on the event rates during the immediate post-insertion period when any real effects of the timing of the insertion would be most apparent.

Postabortal Insertion

Several investigators have evaluated postabortal IUD insertions by comparing the rates of complications which occurred either at the time of postabortal IUD insertion or in the first few weeks after insertion with complication rates of women who had abortions, but no IUD insertions. These studies demonstrate that IUDs may be inserted immediately after abortion without increased risks to the patients.

Goldsmith and co-workers (12) inserted Lippes Loops D in 295 postabortal women and also evaluated 289 postabortal women who did not receive an

Table 2.1 Rates of various complications within eight weeks of a first trimester-induced abortion.

Complication	Abortion N = 436 (%)	Abortion and Cu-T Insertion N = 196 (%)
Bleeding requiring transfusion or repeat curettage	3.7	3.6
Cervical laceration with suture, suspected or confirmed uterine perforation	0.5	0.0
Temperature $\geq$ 38C for $\geq$ 1 day	2.1	0.0
Pathologic findings at follow-up examination	6.9	6.1
Increased blood sedimentation rate of $\geq$ 5 mm above preabortion rate in cases of suspected infection	6.2	3.6
Hospital readmission	6.0	3.1

Source: Adapted from Nygren, K. D., and Johansson, E. D. B. (27)

IUD in a double-blind study where all the women believed they had an IUD in situ. By the one month follow-up visit, no statistically significant differences were found between the two groups of women with respect to frequency of medications prescribed, days of antibiotic use, degree of fever with or without antibiotics, amount of bleeding or pain after currettage, duration or amount of bleeding, pain or abnormal gynecological findings.

Nygren and Johansson (27) found no significant difference in the rates of somatic complications which occurred eight weeks after the insertion of Cu-T IUDs in 196 women immediately following first trimester induced abortions compared to a control group of 436 women who received abortions but no IUD insertions (Table 2.1).

Hue and co-workers (18) compared the outcome of 1,104 women who had first or second trimester induced abortions followed by Lippes Loop insertions and 1,124 patients who had abortions but no IUD insertions. Significantly higher rates of back pain and leukorrhea were recorded for the women who received IUDs, but no significant differences were found in the rates of postabortal infection, bleeding or spotting.

Larsson and Hamberger (22) also evaluated complication rates after insertion of Cu-7 IUDs in 43 patients who aborted at 6 to 8 weeks' gestation and in 55 patients who aborted at 8 to 12 weeks' gestation, compared to 100 patients who aborted at 6 to 8 weeks' gestation and 541 patients who aborted at 8 to 12 weeks' gestation who had no IUD insertions. At routine gynecological examination 10 to 14 days after discharge, the rates of suspicious and manifest infections were significantly lower for the Cu-7 and abortion groups than for the abortion only group. Rates of recurettage were similar for the two groups.

Solheim and Rydnert (35) measured uterine blood loss in 143 women who had copper-bearing IUDs inserted immediately after a first trimester abortion and contrasted this with the findings among 163 women who had no IUD inserted after their abortions. No significant differences were found in the mean blood loss of the two groups of women within four hours after completion of the abortion or within the first seven days after the abortion.

Burkman and co-workers (8) conducted a case-control study to evaluate the risks of postabortal endometritis within the one month following elective abortion and immediate insertion of the Lippes Loop or Dalkon Shield. They found no increased risks, and perhaps a decreased risk, of postabortal endometritis among those women who had an IUD inserted compared to their matched controls (those who had an abortion but no IUD insertion). Furthermore, there was no significant difference in the rates of postabortal endometritis between the Lippes Loop and the Dalkon Shield acceptors.

Postpartum Insertion

IUDs which are inserted either immediately after delivery or during the puerperium have a higher expulsion rate than do IUDs which are inserted after complete uterine involution. IUD expulsion rates for postpartum insertions from various studies are summarized in Table 2.2. The variations in expulsion rates probably reflect differences in the insertion techniques used, the timing of the insertions and the durations of follow-up.

High rates of IUD expulsion during the puerperium may be expected since the uterus is involuting during this period and the contracting uterus generally expels retained placenta, blood clots and other debris. Few IUDs have been designed for retention by the enlarged postpartum uterus. The mechanisms by which IUDs are retained in the nonpuerperal uterus are probably ineffective when IUDs are inserted postpartum. The addition of biodegradable extensions in either the anterior-posterior direction or the lateral plane of the uterus have been proposed as a solution to the high expulsion rates associated with postpartum IUD insertions. Such extensions would be designed to degrade at a controlled rate that would conform to the usual rate of uterine involution. Prototypes of devices specifically designed for postpartum insertion are currently being evaluated in clinical field trials (19).

Two potentially serious complications which occur in association with postpartum IUD insertions are uterine perforation and infection. These are discussed in detail in Chapters 3 and 4.

Complications at the Time of IUD Insertion

Uterine perforation is a major complication of IUD insertion. The intrauterine sound, the inserter and the IUD all have been implicated as causes of per-

Table 2.2 Expulsion rates for postpartum IUD insertions.

Reference Number	IUD	Insertions (Number)	Time of Insertion	Expulsion Rate
24	Lippes Loop Saf-T-Coil Birnberg Bow	788 72 39	Before hospital discharge; 93% 2–3 days postpartum	20.0% within 6 months; 8% within 2 days
28	Lippes Loop	719	Not stated	37.8% within 3 months
5	Lippes Loop	7,122	Before hospital discharge; 93.8% before 10 days postpartum	19.0/100 women at 1-year (net life-table rate)
10	Lippes Loop	400	4–8 days postpartum	26.4% of women followed within 6 weeks
6	Lippes Loop	268	After delivery of placenta	4.4% of women followed within 1 month
20	Cu-T-200	197	2–18 days postpartum; 90.8% before 8 days postpartum	10.9/100 women within 3 months; 14.8/100 women at 1 year (net life-table rates)
39	Lippes Loop Dalkon Shield	633 407	56% Dalkon Shields, 90% Lippes Loops within 3 days postpartum. All within 6 weeks of delivery	Lippes Loop: 1.7/100 women within 1 month; 3.5/100 women within 3 months. Dalkon Shield: 4.1/100 women within 1 month; 8.3/women within 3 months (net life-table rates)
26	Lem Cu-7 Progestasert	100 123 51	After delivery of placenta	At 6 weeks postpartum: Lem—7.0%; Cu-7—7.3%; Progestasert—2.0%

foration (see Chapter 3). Far more common than perforation is the inability to insert the IUD successfully. Unfortunately, this complication is frequently overlooked or not reported, so that the actual incidence of failed insertion is difficult to determine.

Preparations for Insertion

The patient must be able to relax sufficiently to permit a careful bimanual examination, speculum insertion and intravaginal instrument manipulation. If she is unable to cooperate in this manner, it is unwise to proceed. In selected instances, premedication with a mild tranquilizer (5–10 mg of diazepam) may be helpful. Of greater importance is the pre-insertion counseling provided the patient which should include a complete explanation of the insertion procedure.

The amount of cervical dilatation required for IUD insertion depends on the size of the IUD and the condition of the cervix. If cervical dilatation is required, it is advisable to administer intracervical or paracervical block anesthesia. The need for such local anesthesia can be assessed at the time of pelvic examination and uterine sounding. If the woman experiences significant pain during this procedure, local anesthesia is advised. Five to ten milliliters of a 1% solution of xylocaine with or without epinephrine (1:200,000) may be injected under the mucosal surface at the three and nine o'clock positions of the cervix.

Difficult Insertions

The frequency of difficult IUD insertions varies with the type of IUD, the parity of the patient and the skill of the operator. Numerous studies have documented a higher incidence of insertion difficulties among nulliparas as compared to multiparas, though their exact nature is usually not stated.

Rates of difficult insertions for the Cu-T given by Landesman and co-workers (21) were 9.1% for nulligravidas (143 attempted insertions) and 1.0% for multigravidas (199 attempted insertions). Moreover, the Cu-T could not be inserted in six (4.0%) nulligravidas while no such difficulties were observed in multigravidas.

Zador and co-workers (41) reported difficulties in the insertion of the Progestasert in 17.1% of 35 nulliparas compared to 1.7% of 115 multiparas.

Ros (31) experienced insertion difficulties with the standard size Dalkon Shield in 8.3% of 24 milliparas and 1.3% of 150 multiparas. Rates of insertion difficulties for 71 nulliparas and 73 multiparas who had Cu-7, Cu-T or Progestasert IUDs inserted were 2.8% and 5.5%, respectively.

Severe or Persistent Pain

Patients occasionally develop severe or persistent pain moments after IUD insertion and may request immediate removal of the device.

Willson and co-workers (40) reported removal for severe cramping during the first postinsertion day from four (0.6%) of 704 women who had Lippes Loops inserted.

Holtzhausen (15) evaluated 86 Margulies Spiral insertions and 174 Lippes Loop insertions. Two patients had severe vasovagal reactions following the IUD insertion and required immediate IUD removal.

Howard (17) removed Lippes Loops (A, B or C) from seven (4.2%) of 167 nulliparous women for pain and collapse. Postinsertion shock was more pronounced in those patients who had been taking oral contraceptives. No cases of collapse occurred after the oral administration of 10 mg diazepam to women who were tense, apprehensive, amenorrheic or users of oral contraceptives.

In an evaluation of the Dalkon Shield, immediate removal was necessary for two (0.8%) of 256 nulliparous women (16). One patient had a grand mal seizure; the other had severe pain.

Marshall and co-workers (25) reported 18 (6.1%) removals within the first 24 hours following the insertion of Dalkon Shields into 296 nulliparous patients.

Among 400 Cu-T insertions and 400 Cu-7 insertions, immediate removal was necessary for only one patient who had syncope during the insertion of a Cu-7 (33).

Berger and co-workers (7) reported a removal for severe pain immediately after the insertion of a Lippes Loop B in one of 27 nulliparas.

Changes in Vital Signs

Several investigators have documented changes in vital signs during or immediately following IUD insertion.

Acker and co-workers (2) studied ECG records taken during 87 IUD insertion procedures (Lippes Loop D, 78 cases; Loop A, four cases, Dalkon Shield, five cases). There were no significant changes in 58 (66.7%) patients. Eight (9.2%) women demonstrated sustained tachycardia at rest, during insertion and five minutes after insertion. Ten (11.5%) patients had tachycardia during the procedure, and 11 patients (12.6%) had bradycardia or arrhythmia upon IUD insertion. Acker and co-workers (2) also reported on one woman with a history of previous syncopal episodes who sustained a cardiac arrest following an IUD insertion. The woman responded immediately to intravenous administration of 0.4 mg atropine sulfate.

Sherrod and Nicholl (34) also evaluated changes in the cardiac rate which were documented by ECG recordings among 24 nulligravidas and one multipara, each of whom had a standard-size Dalkon Shield inserted. Introduction of the metal speculum or application of the tenaculum produced no significant changes. During uterine sounding, six (24%) patients experienced significant increases in heart rate, while 14 (56%) showed significant decreases in heart rate. Five women (20%) had sinus tachycardia, and eight (32%) had sinus bradycardia. Similar reactions were observed during insertion of the IUD: increased heart rate in 28%, with sinus tachycardia in 20%; decreased heart rate in 56%, with sinus bradycardia in 28%.

Aznar and co-workers (4) studied the cardiac changes which occurred during 50 Lippes Loop, 54 Progestasert, 50 Cu-T and 50 Cu-7 insertions, and during 31 endometrial biopsy and seven uterine lavage procedures. Bradycardia or tachycardia occurred significantly more often with the Lippes Loop and Cu-7 insertions (62.0%) than they did with either the Progestasert of the Cu-T insertions (35.6%) or with the other intrauterine procedures (42.9%). However, the severity of the bradycardia or tachycardia was similar for all groups of patients.

Berger and co-workers (7) evaluated 93 nulligravid women undergoing IUD insertion (Lippes Loop A, 27; Dalkon Shield, 28; Cu-7, 38). Changes in systolic or diastolic blood pressure of 10 or more mmHg, in the pulse rate of 10 or more beats per minute and in the respiration rate of three or more respirations per minute were frequently observed two to five minutes after the IUD insertion compared to values at the preinsertion physical examination.

These studies do not consistently demonstrate specific changes in vital signs to be associated with any
particular device. Since changes in cardiac rate have
been observed by Sherrod and Nicholl (34) during
uterine sounding, as well as during IUD insertion, it
is most likely that the effects on the cardiac system
that occur during IUD insertion are due to neuro-
genic stimuli which arise from cervical manipulation and/or dilation or from the sensation of pain.

Vasovagal Reactions

Many patients experience vasovagal signs and
symptoms (pallor, diaphoresis, bradycardia, hypo-
tension and weakness) during or immediately after
the IUD insertion. These side effects are usually
mild and transient and do not warrant immediate
removal of the IUD. When they are severe or persistent, the intravenous injection of 0.4 mg atropine
sulfate usually affords prompt relief.
     The incidence of vasovagal reactions for specific
IUDs cannot be determined adequately from the published literature. The proper selection of patients,
the amount of cervical manipulation and/or dilation
required, as well as the skill of the person who inserts the IUD all probably affect the occurrence of
these reactions. Some clinicians contend that the
prophylactic administration of paracervical block
anesthesia may prevent vasovagal reactions, but this
has not been documented in any published study.

Seizures

Grand mal seizures occur rarely in association with
IUD insertion or removal. To our knowledge, only 12
cases have been reported which occurred immediately following the insertion or removal of an IUD.
These are summarized in Table 2.3. Some of the 12

Table 2.3 Case reports of grand mal seizures in association with an IUD insertion or removal.

Reference Number	Case Number	IUD Inserted	Parity	History	Comments
30	—	NS*	NS	NS	2,000 insertions with 5 cases of grand mal seizure immediately following insertion
2	1	NS	3	Syncopal episodes	Seizure shortly after insertion followed by apparent cardiac arrest
9	1	Lippes Loop D	2	Negative	Seizure within minutes of insertion
	2	Lippes Loop (removed)	0	Complicated, including epilepsy	Seizure immediately following removal
	3	Lippes Loop	0	Negative	Seizure during insertion followed by seizure after insertion
16	1	Dalkon Shield	NS	NS	(No comment)
29	1	None	0	Fainting spells	Seizure after sounding the uterus and prior to insertion
	2	Lippes Loop C	4	Negative	Seizure immediately following insertion

* NS = not stated

patients had a history of syncopal episodes which may have placed them at higher risk of grand mal seizure; others did not. In those patients for whom follow-up took place, no subsequent seizures or late ill effects were reported. The true incidence of grand mal seizures associated with IUD insertion is probably less than 0.5% as indicated in the following studies:

> Ringrose (30) reported five seizures in 2,000 insertions (0.25%). Conrad and co-workers (9) noted three seizures in 7,140 insertions (0.04%). Horowitz (16) observed one seizure in 256 insertions (0.4%).

Summary

An IUD can be inserted at any time during the menstrual cycle, as well as postabortion and postpartum, but the expulsion rate is higher after insertions which occur less than six weeks postpartum. No less important than the optimum timing of insertion is the proper selection of patients. A careful evaluation of each patient's medical history as it pertains to the contraindications to IUD use will help eliminate potentially serious complications. The occurrence of uterine perforation in particular will be reduced if cervical stenosis and severe anterior or posterior uterine displacements are accepted as absolute contraindications.

It seems to be clearly established that improved results could be obtained with available IUDs if each woman were able to receive a device of appropriate size. At present, however, there are no decision-making rules to use as a guide in matching individual women and specific devices.

The most frequently reported complications which occur immediately after the IUD is inserted are pain and vasovagal reactions. It is probable that these conditions can be minimized by use of a paracervical block anesthesia and adherence to careful technique. Atropine sulfate should be readily available anytime an IUD is inserted so that it may be used to treat rare but potentially serious vagal reactions.

References

1. A. H. Robins Company. Unpublished data. Richmond, Virginia.

2. Acker, D.; Boehm, F. H.; Askew, D. E.; and Rothman, H. Electrocardiogram changes with intrauterine contraceptive device insertion. *Am. J. Obstet. Gynecol.* 115:458, 1973.

3. Akinla, O.; Luukkainen, T.; and Timonen, H. Important factors in the use-effectiveness of the Copper-T-200 IUD. *Contraception* 12:697, 1975.

4. Aznar, R.; Reynoso, L.; Ley, E.; Gamez, R.; and De Leon, M.D. Electrocardiographic changes induced by insertion of an intrauterine device and other uterine manipulations. *Fertil. Steril.* 27:93, 1976.

5. Banharnsupawat, L., and Rosenfield, A. G. Immediate postpartum IUD insertion. *Obstet. Gynecol.* 38:276, 1971.

6. Baveja, R., and Samant, V. Immediate postpartum Lippes Loop insertion "a short term trial." *J. Obstet. Gynaecol.* (India) XXIV:165, 1974.

7. Berger, G. S.; Edelman, D. A.; and Regenie, S. J. Patients' responses to IUD insertion. *Int. J. Gynaecol. Obstet.* 14:146, 1976.

8. Burkman, R. T.; Tonascia, J. A.; Atienza, M. F.; and King, T. M. The relationship of immediate post-abortal intrauterine device insertion to subsequent endometritis: a case-control study. *Contraception* 15:435, 1977.

9. Conrad, C. C.; Ghazi, M.; and Kitay, D. Z. Acute neuro-vascular sequelae of intrauterine device insertion or removal. *J. Reprod. Med.* 11:211, 1973.

10. Engineer, A. D., and Sanwal, K. A comparative study of postpartum, puerperal, and non-puerperal insertions of Lippes Loops. *J. Obstet. Gynaecol.* (India) XXII:262, 1972.

11. Esposito, J. M.; Zarou, D. M.; and Zarou, G. S. A Dalkon Shield imbedded in a myoma: case report of an unusual displacement of an intrauterine contraceptive device. *Am. J. Obstet. Gynecol.* 117:578, 1973.

12. Goldsmith, A.; Goldberg, R.; Eyzaguirre, H.; Lucero, S.; and Lizana, L. IUD insertion in the immediate post-abortal period. In *Family planning research conference, a multi-disciplinary approach*, eds. A. Goldsmith, and R. Snowden, Amsterdam: Excerpta Medica, 1972.

13. Hallatt, J. G. Repeat ectopic pregnancy: a study of 123 consecutive cases. *Am. J. Obstet. Gynecol.* 122:520, 1975.

14. Hasson, H. M.; Berger, G. S.; and Edelman, D. A. Factors affecting intrauterine contraceptive device performance I. Endometrial cavity length. *Am. J. Obstet. Gynecol.* 126:973, 1976.

15. Holtzhausen, G. H. R. Preliminary report on the use of intra-uterine contraception in private practice. *S. A. J. Obstet. Gynecol.* 6:18, 1967.

16. Horowitz, A. J. A study of contraceptive effectiveness and incidence of side effects with the use of the Dalkon Shield. *Contraception* 7:1, 1973.

17. Howard, G. Use of intrauterine devices in nulliparous women. *Lancet* 2:1339, 1972.

18. Hue, K.; Kwon, H. Y.; Michael, P. H.; and Watson, W. B. A comparative study of the safety and efficacy of

postabortal intrauterine contraceptive device insertion. *Am. J. Obstet. Gynecol.* 118:975, 1974.

19. International Fertility Research Program. Unpublished data. Research Triangle Park, North Carolina.

20. Laes, E.; Lehtovirta, P.; Weintraub, D.; Pyorala, T.; and Luukkainen, T. Early puerperal insertions of Copper-T-200. *Contraception* 11:289, 1975.

21. Landesman, R.; Kaye, R. E.; and Wilson, K. H. A two-man experience with the Copper "T" intrauterine device. *Contraception* 7:477, 1973.

22. Larsson, B., and Hamberger, L. Insertion of Copper-7 IUDs in connection with induced abortions during the first trimester. *Contraception* 12:69, 1975.

23. Lippes, J.; Malik, T.; and Tatum, H. J. The post-coital Copper-T. *Adv. Plann. Parent.* XI:24, 1976.

24. London, G. D., and Anderson, G. V. Immediate post-partum insertion of an intrauterine contraceptive device. *Obstet. Gynecol.* 30:851, 1967.

25. Marshall, B. R.; Hepler, J. K.; Scott, R. H.; and Zirbel, C. C. The Dalkon Shield in nulliparous women. *Am. J. Obstet. Gynecol.* 118:186, 1974.

26. Newton, J.; Harper, M.; and Chan, K. K. Immediate post-placental insertion of intrauterine contraceptive devices. *Lancet* 2:272, 1977.

27. Nygren, K-G., and Johansson, E. D. B. Insertion of the endouterine Copper-T (TCu-200) immediately after first trimester legal abortion. *Contraception* 7:299, 1973.

28. Phatak, L. V., and Bhatia, M. Observations on expulsion of the IUCD in puerperal and nonpuerperal insertions. *Am. J. Obstet. Gynecol.* 101:773, 1968.

29. Richardson, J.; Morrison, J.; Chang, A.; and Morri-

son, J. Epileptiform convulsions during insertion of intrauterine contraceptive device. *Lancet* 2:148, 1977.

30. Ringrose, C. Intrauterine contraceptive devices. *J. Reprod. Med.* 6:96, 1971.

31. Ros, A. Our experience with the use of five different medicated intrauterine devices. *Contraception* 4:271, 1977.

32. Schoen, J. A., and Nowak, R. J. Repeat ectopic pregnancy: a 116-year clinical survey. *Obstet. Gynecol.* 45:542, 1975.

33. Shaila, N. G.; Lane, M. E.; and Sobrero, A. J. A comparative randomized double-blind study of the Copper-T-200 and Copper-7 intrauterine contraceptive devices with modified insertion techniques. *Am. J. Obstet. Gynecol.* 120:110, 1974.

34. Sherrod, D. B., and Nicholl, W. Electrocardiographic changes during intrauterine contraceptive device insertion. *Am. J. Obstet. Gynecol.* 119:1044, 1974.

35. Solheim, F., and Rydnert, J. Vacuum aspiration at therapeutic abortion—effect of Cu-IUD insertion at operation on post-operative blood loss. *Contraception* 13:707, 1976.

36. Tejuja, S., and Malkani, P. K. Clinical significance of correlation between size of uterine cavity and IUCD. A study by planimeter-hysterogram technique. *Am. J. Obstet. Gynecol.* 105:620, 1969.

37. Vago, T., and Spira, H. Pregnancy in a bicornuate uterus after insertion of a Lippes Loop (on the horns of a dilemma). *Am. J. Obstet. Gynecol.* 97:872, 1967.

38. Wheeler, R.; Buschbom, R. L.; and Marshall, R. K. Rational basis for IUD design and development. In *Intrauterine devices: development, evaluation, and program implementation*, eds. R. G. Wheeler, G. W. Dun-

can, and J. J. Speidel. New York: Academic Press, 1974.

39. Wiknjosastro, H.; Doodoh, A.; Rachman, I. A.; Aguss-jaries, Harap H.; Mitra, M.; and Thomas, M. Postpartum use of the Lippes Loop and Dalkon Shield. In *Proceedings of the Asian Federation of Obstetrics and Gynecology, 1st Inter-Congress*, Vol. 2, ed. S. M. M. Karim. Singapore, 1976.

40. Willson, J. R.; Ledger, W. J.; and Lovell, J. Intrauterine contraceptive devices: a comparison between their use in indigent and private patients. *Obstet. Gynecol.* 29:59, 1967.

41. Zador, G.; Nillson, B. A.; Nillson, B.; Sjoberg, N. O.; Westrom, L.; and Wiese, J. Clinical experience with the uterine progesterone system (Progestasert). *Contraception* 13:559, 1976.

Chapter 3

Uterine perforation

Introduction

Uterine perforation has long been recognized as one of the complications which may accompany the use of IUDs. In the 1930s, both Murphy (65) and Andrews (3) published case reports of perforations with the Gräfenberg ring. Hundreds of cases of uterine perforation have been reported since then and every device in clinical use has been implicated.

Various authors have reviewed the literature pertaining to IUD-related uterine perforation and have enumerated the reported cases of uterine perforation for each type of IUD. These reviews are incomplete because they do not include estimates of the incidence of perforation for each type of IUD. This chapter will provide such estimates and will evaluate the following factors which affect the incidence of perforation: IUD characteristics, patient characteristics, insertion technique, skill and experience of the person who inserts the IUD and the timing of insertion relative to prior pregnancy. Finally, the sequelae of IUD-related uterine perforations and the management of these perforations are discussed.

Definitions

Uterine perforation is defined in this chapter as penetration of the IUD through the wall of the uterine corpus; cervical perforation refers to IUD penetration through the uterine cervix. Uterine perforations are defined as complete if the IUD has completely passed through the uterine wall and partial if part of the IUD is still within the uterus or myometrium. The term "perforation" does not include embedment of the IUD into the myometrium. Primary perforations are those which occur at the time of IUD insertion, and secondary perforations are those which occur after the IUD has been inserted. These differences will be specified whenever possible, but it must be noted that much of the reviewed literature did not provide information about the type, degree or time of perforation.

Incidence of Uterine Perforation

The incidence of uterine perforation commonly quoted in the literature varies widely with the type of IUD. The Cu-T is at the low end of the spectrum with a perforation rate of 0.2 per 1,000 insertions, or one out of 5,000 insertions (90,105). The rate progresses to 0.4 per 1,000 insertions, or one out of 2,500 insertions for the Lippes Loop (63,91,94). The Dalkon Shield is at the upper end of the spectrum with a perforation rate of 2.9 per 1,000 insertions, or one in 350 insertions (41,63). Careful review of the literature, however, does not support the accuracy of these figures since reported perforation rates for each type of IUD are considerably different from those which are most often quoted. For example, the commonly quoted uterine perforation rate of one per 350 Dalkon Shield insertions is based on a study by Snowden and Williams (99) who reported three perforations in the first 1,031 insertions performed during the University of Exeter's Family Planning Research Unit multiclinic evaluation. In a subsequent report on this evaluation, the uterine perfora-

Table 3.1 The incidence of cervical and uterine perforations for interval IUD insertions.

IUD	Number of Insertions	Cervical Perforations Number	Cervical Perforations Rate/1000	Uterine Perforations Number	Uterine Perforations Rate/1000
Antigon	8,605	0	0.0	1	0.1
Birnberg Bow	7,193	0	0.0	69	9.6
Cu-T	20,066	30	1.5	5	0.3
Cu-7	22,914	4	0.2	14	0.6
Dalkon Shield	29,285	0	0.0	42	1.4
Lippes Loop*	277,300	0	0.0	35	0.1
Lippes Loop†	76,631	0	0.0	89	1.2
Margulies Spiral	5,675	12	2.1	6	1.1
Progestasert	11,389	8	0.7	5	0.4
Saf-T-Coil	4,122	0	0.0	0	0.0
Ypsilon	3,822	0	0.0	0	0.0

* SOURCE: Liao et al. (56), study based on a mail survey
† SOURCE: All other Lippes Loop studies, excluding Liao et al. (56)

tion rate fell to 0.8 per 1,000 insertions, based on five perforations in 6,070 insertions (26). Thus, when the first 1,031 insertions were excluded, the perforation rate had declined to only 0.4 per 1,000 insertions, or about one in 2,500.

Table 3.1 presents estimates of the incidence of cervical and uterine perforation for interval insertions (i.e., insertions performed at least two months after delivery or at least one month after abortion) for the following IUDs: Antigon, Birnberg Bow, Cu-T, Cu-7, Dalkon Shield, Lippes Loop, Margulies Spiral, Progestasert, Saf-T-Coil and Ypsilon. These estimates are based on data derived from numerous literature reports; multiple reports of identical cases have been excluded whenever possible. The numbers of puerperal insertions for any specific IUDs could not always be identified in each published report; thus, the perforation rates given in Table 3.1 should be considered approximate. Listed in appendix A are some studies which have reported on perforation rates for various types of IUDs.

The Birnberg Bow is observed to have a higher perforation rate than the other devices, but all the remaining IUDs share similar lower rates. Cervical perforation rates are higher for the Cu-T, Progestasert and Margulies Spiral than they are for the other IUDs. Two estimates of the perforation rate for the Lippes Loop are given in Table 3.1; one is based on the mail survey conducted by Liao and co-workers (56) which probably underestimated the actual perforation rates, and the other is based on all other studies.

A national mail survey conducted in June 1973 by the National Center for Disease Control (CDC) to estimate IUD-related morbidity serious enough to require hospitalization provides additional evidence for the lack of significant differences in the incidence of uterine perforation for different types of IUDs.

An analysis of the CDC survey data was conducted to evaluate the association between the use of the Dalkon Shield and subsequent hospitalization for complicated pregnancies (45). It was found that 22.7%, 27.9% and 24.5%, respectively, of hospitalized users of the Dalkon Shield, Lippes Loop and Saf-T-Coil were admitted with a diagnosis of uterine perforation. Moreover, the rates of hospitalization for uterine perforation for the Dalkon Shield and the Saf-T-Coil users were not significantly different (p>.10), but were significantly lower (p<.05) than the hospitalization rate for the Lippes Loop users.

In another analysis of the CDC data, Mosley, Chow and Lui (64) concluded that the total hospitalization rate, when adjusted for duration of IUD use, for the Dalkon Shield user was 4 to 18% higher than the rate for the Lippes Loop or Saf-T-Coil users. If the data presented by Kahn and Tyler (45) are adjusted to reflect the increased hospitalization rate for the Dalkon Shield users, then the adjusted hospitalization rates for uterine perforation for Dalkon Shield users ranges from 23.7 to 27.7%. The rates for the Saf-T-Coil and Lippes Loop users are 24.5 and 27.9%,

respectively. These rates are not significantly different (p>.10) from those for the Dalkon Shield. It is
interesting to note that the 325 Dalkon Shield users
who were hospitalized with a diagnosis of uterine
perforation represented 40.9% of all hospitalized
uterine perforation patients reported by Kahn and
Tyler (45). The Dalkon Shield has been estimated to
account for about 40% of all IUD sales in the United
States for the period covered by the Kahn and Tyler
study.

The perforation rates presented in Table I should
be considered a lower limit of the true incidence of
uterine perforations. Careful follow-up and meticulous examination of all patients may lead to the reporting of higher rates of perforation.

In an evaluation of the Birnberg Bow, three perforations were discovered among the first 544 insertions
(10). Further use of the Bow was abandoned by the
investigator. Careful examination of the remaining
541 patients who had a Bow inserted led to the diagnosis of an additional 13 perforations, or a perforation rate of 29.4 per 1,000 (544 insertions) compared
to 2.7 per 1,000 (751 insertions) for the Lippes Loop.
    Ratnam and Tow (79) reported a perforation rate
of 10.4 per 1,000 (93 perforations in 8,977 insertions)
for the Lippes Loop. This rate is considerably higher
than those reported by other investigators. Ratnam
and Tow's study, however, was designed specifically
to investigate the possibility of uterine perforation.

Most other reported studies generally do not provide
specific data regarding patient follow-up, the criteria
for initiating an investigation for possible uterine
perforation or the diagnostic techniques used to investigate a possible perforation. Therefore, it is not
possible to calculate the true incidence of uterine
perforation for various types of IUDs.

Diagnosis of Uterine Perforation

Disagreement as to when uterine perforations occur
has not been resolved. Although uterine perforations
may occur at the time of IUD insertion or subsequent
to the insertion, the relative frequency of these two
events for various IUDs remains unknown. Hall (34),
for example, is of the opinion that all uterine perforations occur at insertion. Other investigators dis-
agree (6,12,13,79). Evidence that some uterine perforations may occur after IUD insertion has been
provided by Ratnam and Tow (79) who reported
three cases where the tailed end of a Lippes Loop
had perforated the uterus while the rest of the IUD
lay within the endometrial cavity. If the perforation
had occurred at the time of insertion, it would be
reasonable to expect that the leading end of the IUD
would have protruded through the uterine wall. The
fact that the tailed end had perforated the uterus
suggests that either an intrauterine repositioning of
the IUD had taken place or that downward expulsive
forces had caused the tail to become embedded in
the myometrium through which it ultimately protruded.

Since most uterine perforations are not diagnosed
at the time of IUD insertion, the true incidence of
uterine perforation cannot be assessed accurately
unless all subjects are seen periodically and evaluated for the presence of the IUD in the endometrial
cavity.

> Liao and co-workers (56) reported that only 6 (22.2%)
> of 27 uterine perforations were diagnosed at the time
> of insertion, and that the diagnosis of perforation
> was made more than six months after insertion in
> 40.7% of patients wearing Lippes Loops.
>
> Ratnam and Tow (79) found that 58.1% of 93
> uterine perforations by Lippes Loops were not diag-
> nosed until seven or more months after the inser-
> tions.

Table 3.2 *Proportions of asymptomatic patients at the time of diagnosed uterine perforation.*

Reference Number	Number of Patients	Percentage Asymptomatic Patients
34	19	100.0
119	14	85.7
56	35	71.4
79	93	100.0
101	63	38.2
32	31	58.1

Signs and symptoms which suggest uterine perforation at IUD insertion may include difficulty in inserting the IUD as well as pain and bleeding which occur at insertion or immediately thereafter. Pain and bleeding are frequent responses to the insertion of any IUD and also represent the most frequent medical reasons for IUD removal. Thus, in many cases, patients with uterine perforations may have symptoms which are not specific to perforation, or they may be totally asymptomatic (Table 3.2).

Many perforations are asymptomatic, and neither the patient nor the physician may have reason to suspect the presence of an extrauterine IUD. In these instances, the patient is not protected from pregnancy; in fact, pregnancy may be the first sign which suggests the possibility of an extrauterine IUD.

In the series of 93 perforations reported by Ratnam and Tow (79), 28 (30.1%) patients were pregnant at the time of diagnosis of the uterine perforation. Pregnancy led to the diagnosis of uterine perforation in 4 (28.6%) of 14 cases reported by Wei (119), 3 (23.1%) of 13 cases reported by Whitson and co-workers (120), 16 (84.2%) of 19 cases reported by Hall (34) and 5 (7.9%) of 63 cases reported by Somboonsuk and co-workers (101).

Table 3.3 Incidence of uterine perforation for patients with "missing" IUD strings.

Reference Number	Number of Patients with Missing Strings	Uterine Perforations	
		Number	Percentage
81	25	0	0.0
20	45	8	17.8
67	40	0	0.0
39	55	2	3.6
4	9	5	55.6
43	44	0	0.0
93	21	3	14.3
118	91	6	6.6

Uterine perforation is frequently diagnosed when the IUD strings are missing (Table 3.3), but failure to see the strings at the external cervical os does not necessarily imply that the IUD has been expelled or is in an extrauterine location. Conversely, IUD strings which are visible at the external cervical os do not guarantee that the device is in the uterine cavity.

Valle and co-workers (116,117,118) have used the hysteroscope for the evaluation of IUD users with missing IUD strings. They found the IUD within the uterine cavity in 78 of the 91 cases studied (118). In the remaining 13 patients, no IUD was found within the uterine cavity. In six of the latter patients, the IUD was shown radiographically to be in an extrauterine location.

Among the 93 uterine perforations reported by Ratnam and Tow (79), the strings of the Lippes Loop were visible at the cervical os for 46 (50.5%) cases when the diagnosis of uterine perforation was made. The diagnosis was suspected in some of these cases because either the IUD strings were retracted into the cervix or traction on the strings failed to dislodge the IUD.

Whenever the diagnosis of uterine perforation is suspected, vaginal and rectovaginal examinations should be performed. Palpation of the anterior or posterior uterine surface may reveal abnormalities which indicate an extrauterine device. Occasionally, the IUD may be felt in the posterior cul-de-sac (31, 42,89). If the device is not located on physical examination of a nonpregnant patient, the uterus may be probed with a sound (96) or an IUD hook (51,93) to detect and remove a device which is located within the uterine cavity. Alternatively, x-ray examination may be used. Plain x-ray examination of the abdomen is useful in demonstrating the presence of an IUD, but the diagnosis of perforation can be made with a plain film only if the IUD is located outside the pelvis (112,113). Flat-plate and lateral pelvic x-ray by themselves are often unable to distinguish between an intrauterine location and a perforating IUD (28,109). Manipulating the uterus under fluoroscopic examination or the introduction of an intrauterine marker, such as a uterine sound, will help to determine whether an IUD is intra- or extrauterine (4,21). Other radiographic procedures that can identify the intrauterine cavity and then discriminate between an intrauterine or extrauterine IUD include the intrauterine insertion of a Foley catheter containing radiopaque material and hysterography or hysterosalpingography (20,46,47,112). The insertion of a second IUD as an intrauterine marker has also been advocated prior to radiologic examination for location of a lost IUD (113). Although all of these procedures help to determine whether an IUD is inside or outside the uterus, they are contraindicated during known or suspected pregnancy. The diagnosis of pregnancy must be considered whenever a patient presents with a "lost" IUD.

Winters (123) first reported on the use of ultrasound to locate the IUD. More recent efforts have used the compound B-scanning technique (16,18,39, 40,43,67,75,78,124).

Ianniruberto and Mastroberardino (39) used ultrasound to determine the location of the IUD in 55 patients with missing strings. The location of the missing IUD by ultrasound was correct in all cases, including two cases of uterine perforation (one partial and one complete).

Janssens and co-workers (40) reported that ultrasound correctly identified the IUD in 98% of 110 women known to have had a Lippes Loop inserted. Among 110 women in whom the type of IUD inserted was unknown, ultrasonic detection proved to be correct in only 89% of the cases.

Eyck and co-workers (25), using the improved grey-scale sonography, correctly identified and located six types of IUDs in a series of 58 women.

McArdle (60) used ultrasound and correctly diagnosed the presence or absence of the missing IUD in 50 of 51 patients, including three patients in whom the IUD had perforated the uterus.

Although ultrasound avoids x-ray irradiation of the uterus for a possibly pregnant patient, several investigators (39,40,43) have cautioned that ultrasound may fail to locate an intrauterine IUD when the patient is pregnant. These reports are in contrast to that of Tsai and co-workers (114) who reported 11 cases of successful localization of intrauterine IUDs during pregnancy.

The Beolocator, a device designed to detect metallic and nonmetallic foreign bodies in human tissue has also been used to determine the location of an IUD (29,81). Jouppila (43) evaluated both the Beolocator and the ultrasonic B-scanning technique and found the latter to be a more reliable method for locating the missing IUD. The Beolocator is no longer manufactured and does not appear to be in popular use.

Factors Related to Perforation

Differences in the reported uterine perforation rates may reflect a number of factors which predispose IUD users to uterine perforation; among these are: uterine size and position, cervical stenosis, uterine consistency, cervical or uterine anomalies, inherent IUD design, inserter rigidity and perhaps most important, physician experience. Factors most frequently reported in the literature include: timing of the insertion, physician experience, and insertion technique. These factors are often interrelated; unfortunately, existing reports generally do not permit assessment of the interrelationships of these factors.

Timing of the Insertion

The risk of uterine perforation is increased when an IUD is inserted in the postpartum period. The risk appears to be higher for the IUDs inserted four to eight weeks postpartum than for any other time period.

Tietze (110) reported a perforation rate of 34 per 1,000 insertions with the Birnberg Bow when it was inserted before the sixth postpartum week. This rate declined to 2 per 1,000 when the Bow was inserted after the twelfth postpartum week.

Lean (52) found a higher perforation rate for the Lippes Loop when it was inserted four to six weeks postpartum (11.8 per 1,000) than when it was inserted within one week postpartum (0.9 per 1,000) or eight weeks postpartum (5.8 per 1,000).

Ratnam and Tow (79) reported perforation rates of 2.4, 0.0, 18.3 and 4.2 per 1,000 insertions of the Lippes Loop when it was inserted 48 hours or less, 48 hours to four weeks, four to eight weeks, and eight or more weeks postpartum, respectively.

The enlarged postpartum uterus may more easily permit the IUD to become displaced. Any angular or sharp projection of the displaced IUD may gradually penetrate the myometrium and enter the uterine wall as uterine involution occurs. Because of the higher rates of uterine perforation associated with immediate or early puerperal IUD insertion, some physicians have recommended that insertion be delayed until the uterus is fully involuted and the woman has had at least two normal menstrual periods. One investigator (121) suggests that an IUD inserted into the completely involuted uterus is less likely to be expelled or to perforate than an IUD inserted during the postpartum period; moreover, the possibility of displacement is decreased.

The data regarding the risks of uterine perforation for postabortal insertions are less clear. Based on the reports of Hue and co-workers (38), Newton and co-workers (69) and Timonen and Luukkainen (111), there appears to be no increased risk of uterine perforation when IUDs are inserted immediately after a first trimester abortion. These reports contrast with that of Boria and Gordon (9) who report a higher perforation rate for the postabortal insertion of the Dalkon Shield (21.9 per 1,000 based on six perforations in 274 insertions) than for interval insertions of the same IUD (3.7 per 1,000 based on three perforations in 803 insertions).

Experience of the Individual Inserting the IUD

The few reports which have evaluated physician-specific uterine perforation rates indicate that there may be an association between the individual performing the IUD insertion and perforation rates.

Hall (34) reported an interaction between perforation rates, the training of the physician and the type of IUD used:

	Birnberg Bow		Other IUDs	
	Insertions	Perforation Rate/1,000	Insertions	Perforation Rate/1,000
Physician X	338	3.0	875	1.1
Physician Y	415	14.5	1,268	1.6
Resident Z	113	79.6	15	0.0

The perforation rate was highest for resident Z, who had the least experience in inserting the Birnberg Bow. For physician Y it was nearly five times greater than for physician X. The perforation rate with other IUDs was similar for these two physicians.

Out of eight perforations with the Lippes Loop, Scutchfield and Long (89) found that seven were related to one physician who had a perforation rate of 4.3 per 1,000 (1,623 insertions) compared to a rate of 0.2 per 1,000 (4,244 insertions) for all other physicians. In this study, all physicians had specialty training in obstetrics and gynecology.

In a similar analysis of physician-specific IUD perforation rates, Ratnam and Tow (79) derived the following rates of uterine perforation diagnosed at the time of Lippes Loop insertions:

	Insertions	Perforations	Rate/1,000
Dr. X	1,948	12	6.2
Dr. E.	342	1	2.9
Dr. H	429	5	11.7
Dr. W	789	2	2.5
Other doctors	495	0	0.0

All IUD insertions were performed by physicians who had gynecologic experience or who were specially trained to perform IUD insertions, but the physicians with the least gynecologic training (Dr. X, a house officer, and Dr. H, a general practitioner) had higher perforation rates.

Although the person inserting the IUD is an important factor related to the incidence of uterine perforation, training in gynecology is not necessarily the deciding factor. In some programs, paramedical personnel with special training in IUD insertion have been used to insert IUDs without any reported increase in the rate of uterine perforation (8,58,71, 73).

IUD Insertion Technique

The following series of steps are recommended for IUD insertion:

1. bimanual pelvic examination
2. tenaculum stabilization of the cervix to reduce the angulation between the cervical canal and uterine cavity
3. uterine sounding to confirm the position and assess the depth of the uterus, as well as to judge whether the IUD can be passed easily through the cervical canal
4. selection of an IUD appropriate to the size of the endometrial cavity
5. insertion according to the method recommended by the manufacturer, with cervical dilatation if necessary
6. abandonment of the procedure in favor of another type of IUD or another method of contraception if insertion is difficult.

Failure to adhere to these principles is likely to increase the risk of a uterine perforation.

The Singapore program (79) did not require sounding of the uterine cavity or use of a tenaculum to straighten the uterocervical axis. Among 67 of the 93 reported perforations with the Lippes Loop, where the site of perforation was known, 65 (97.0%) occurred through the lower uterine segment. The site of perforation was determined by hysterography or during surgical removal of the IUDs.

Wei (119) found that the site of four (80.0%) of five uterine perforations was located on the uterine wall opposite the direction of uterine flexion.

Hefnawi and co-workers (37) found that 14 (82.4%) of 17 perforations of the posterior uterine wall occurred in anteverted uteri.

In the study by Scutchfield and Long (89), the only apparent difference in the insertion technique among physicians was that the physician who had the highest perforation rate with the Birnberg Bow did not use a uterine sound to determine the length and direction of the uterine cavity prior to the IUD insertion.

Uterine perforation at the time of IUD insertion may occur as a result of a perforation by the IUD inserter even before the IUD is released from it.

The higher incidence of uterine perforation observed with the Birnberg Bow, especially for puerperal insertions, has been attributed in part to the type of inserter used (10,66).

The Alza Corporation (2) reported five uterine and seven cervical perforations among 6,525 insertions with prototype inserters for the Progestasert. After a design change to a flexible, curved inserter with depth indicators to show distance from the external os to the fundus, only one perforation (cervical) occurred among 4,685 insertions.

IUDs are inserted using either the "push" technique, the "withdrawal" technique or a combination of both. When the "push" technique is used, the IUD inserter is introduced into the uterine cavity until it reaches the fundus. The inserter is then pulled back slightly, depending on the size of the IUD, and the IUD is pushed out of the inserter toward the uterine fundus. When the "withdrawal" technique is used, the IUD inserter is introduced into the uterine cavity until it reaches the fundus. The inserter is then totally withdrawn leaving the IUD in the upper uterine segment. The "push" technique is used for insertion of the Lippes Loop and Saf-T-Coil, and the "withdrawal" technique for the insertion of the Cu-T. A combination of these two techniques is used for the Cu-7; the inserter is introduced to the depth of the fundus, the inserter is partially withdrawn and the IUD is then pushed out of the inserter towards the fundus.

The use of the proper IUD insertion technique may reduce both the risk of uterine perforation at the time of insertion, as well as the risk of secondary perforations. Failure to insert the IUD in the correct position may increase the likelihood of IUD displacement; sharp or angular points on the displaced IUD may erode the uterine wall and eventually perforate it.

Johannisson (41) has proposed that there is a lower risk of perforation when the IUD conforms to the size and shape of the uterine cavity. In this regard, the use of a specific measuring device, such as the wing sound, may be appropriate (36). The Anderson Latex Leaf, Ypsilon and Antigon-F are pliant devices and preliminary data which show low rates of uterine perforation support Johannisson's contention (41). Since these devices have not undergone extensive evaluation, however, it is difficult to ascertain whether the design and/or the method of insertion act to minimize the risks of uterine perforation.

IUD Design

IUD design may be related to perforations of the uterine cervix. The Cu-T and Progestasert have higher reported rates of cervical perforation than the Saf-T-Coil, Lippes Loop or Dalkon Shield. Both the Cu-T and Progestasert are T-shaped devices, and most cervical perforations with these devices have occurred when the sharp tip of the vertical arm has penetrated through the uterine wall. Both of these IUDs have been modified to reduce the risks of such perforations.

Sharp or angular parts of an IUD may erode the uterine wall, especially if the IUD is displaced as a result of normal uterine contractions. It is possible that such displacement could result in partial or complete penetration of the IUD through the myometrium and into the peritoneal cavity. On the other hand, these sharp or angular parts are an essential design facet because they reduce the risk of IUD expulsion. Hysterographic studies have shown, for example, that the Cu-T is retained in part because the tips of the transverse arm embed themselves into the endometrium (46,47). The lateral projections of the Dalkon Shield and Multiload IUDs probably are important design features which contribute to the retention of these IUDs, but they may increase the risk of secondary perforations. At present, data are not available either to support or refute this latter hypothesis.

Severe Complications of Extrauterine IUDs

Scott (88) described the results of a mail survey of 6,449 Fellows of the American College of Obstetricians and Gynecologists. The survey identified 192 women who had critical illnesses as a result of complications following uterine perforations. Intestinal obstruction was diagnosed in 15 of these patients (12 with Birnberg Bows, one with a plastic ring and two with unknown types of IUDs). Two deaths were reported, both from amniotic fluid embolism following spontaneous abortion in the second trimester in association with uterine perforation.

Rubin (83) described a case in which a Lippes Loop which had perforated the uterus was removed 1 day after its insertion. Posterior colpotomy drainage was performed 5 days after removal; a subtotal hysterectomy was performed 18 days after removal. The patient died from septic complications 27 days after the Loop removal.

The nationwide mail survey conducted by CDC reported two deaths associated with uterine perforation (44). One woman died from an acute pulmonary embolism and pulmonary infarction nine days after laparotomy for removal of an extrauterine Saf-T-Coil. The second patient died 34 days after colpotomy removal of an extrauterine Lippes Loop. In the second case, autopsy revealed bilateral salpingitis, peritonitis and a recent thromboembolism which occluded the right main pulmonary artery.

Soderstrom (100) reported a case in which an unrecognized intra-abdominal IUD was associated with death. The patient underwent a vaginal hysterectomy and repair of the pelvic floor. A postoperative pelvic abscess occurred and the patient died of sepsis. At autopsy, an IUD was found in the base of the abscess.

In all but one of the above instances, death occurred after the extrauterine IUD had been removed. In some of the cases, it is difficult to differentiate to what extent the patient's death may have been related to the complications directly attributable to the uterine perforation, as opposed to the complications related to the operative procedure undertaken to treat the perforation and resulting complications.

Numerous reports of serious complications which have resulted from either partial or complete uterine perforations have appeared in the literature (Table 3.4). Intestinal obstruction is among the most serious complications which may occur after an IUD perforation. Except for one recent report (17) of bowel obstruction with a Lippes Loop in the presence of acute PID, all cases of intestinal obstruction have been associated with closed devices (Gräfenberg Ring, Birnberg Bow, Antigon, Icon Ring). Shimkin and co-workers (94) postulated that the mechanism of intestinal obstruction is by herniation of a portion of the bowel through the closed device, or by

Table 3.4 Serious complications resulting from uterine perforation.

Complication	IUD	Number of Cases	Reference Number
Bowel Obstruction	Gräfenberg Ring	2	76,84
	Icon Ring	1	19
	Birnberg Bow	19	22,86–88,42,94,108
	Antigon	1	35
	Plastic Ring	1	88
	Unknown	2	88
	Lippes Loop	1	17
Bowel Perforation	Cu-T	1	122
	Lippes Loop	3	17,48,115
	Dalkon Shield	4	1,5,48
	Cu-7	2	12,69
Bladder Perforation	Dalkon Shield	2	4,68
	Lippes Loop	2	83,85
Pelvic Infection	Lippes Loop	4	14,17,77,89
	Dalkon Shield	2	97,120

fixation of the bowel to the IUD by adhesions with subsequent volvulus. The latter mechanism could occur with either open or closed IUDs. Bowel perforations have been associated with the extrauterine, open IUDs such as the Lippes Loop and Dalkon Shield. This complication appears to be rare, since only eight such cases have been reported.

Management of the Extrauterine IUD

The risk of bowel obstruction associated with partial or complete uterine perforations by closed IUDs such as the Birnberg Bow clearly indicates that all closed devices should be removed once the diagnosis of perforation has been made. At present, there does not appear to be agreement as to whether open IUDs such as the Lippes Loop, Saf-T-Coil, Cu-7, Cu-T and Progestasert should be removed from the peritoneal cavity in the absence of symptoms. Some authors (23,24,48,53,82,86) recommend routine re-

moval of open IUDs to avoid the potential risks of
bowel obstruction. Others (57,59) do not advocate
routine removal of open IUDs among asymptomatic
patients.

D'Amico and Israel (17) reported a case of bowel
perforation and subsequent obstruction associated
with an open IUD (Lippes Loop) in a patient with
acute PID; this led them to recommend removal of
any intraperitoneal IUD in patients with acute PID.
It is unlikely that an open extrauterine IUD could be
a direct cause of bowel obstruction; nevertheless, removal of such IUDs may prevent the formation of
intraperitoneal adhesions which may lead to intestinal obstruction.

> Gunaratne and Mahroof (33) described two types of
> adhesion formation associated with extrauterine
> Lippes Loops. One type consisted of adhesions be-
> tween the parallel limbs of the IUD; the other con-
> sisted of adhesions between the IUD and adjacent
> viscera.
>
> On the basis of the histopathological evaluation
> of omentum attached to perforated Lippes Loops in
> five patients, Badawy and Iskander (7) concluded
> that an inflammatory reaction probably occurs in re-
> sponse to the extrauterine IUD.

There is some evidence to suggest that intraperitoneal copper-bearing IUDs cause a more intense
inflammatory reaction than IUDs without copper
(62,104,105,118). For this reason, it has been recommended that all extrauterine copper-bearing IUDs be
removed as soon as the perforation is recognized.
However, the literature indicates that IUDs without
copper also may elicit a peritoneal inflammatory
reaction.

> Ratnam and Yin (80) found no case of pelvic masses
> or abscesses, or dense fibrous reactions among 44
> patients who had an extrauterine Lippes Loop re-

moved. Similar findings have been reported by other investigators (6,30,37,53).

Ansari (4), on the other hand, reported severe local adhesions in association with two or three extrauterine Lippes Loops.

Whitson and co-workers (120) reported that 11 of 13 perforated Dalkon Shields were enveloped in abdominopelvic adhesions. Others (5,48,103) have noted similar findings. However, Ansari (4) and Cederqvist and co-workers (13) noted minimal or no inflammatory reaction to the extrauterine Dalkon Shield. Soderstrom (100) observed that adhesions were associated with 14 (51.9%) of 27 extrauterine Dalkon Shields and with 12 (60.0%) of 20 Lippes Loops. The degree of peritoneal response to the extrauterine IUDs was not reported.

In some cases, the inflammatory response to extrauterine IUDs may be secondary to bacterial contamination which may occur at the time of insertion or subsequent to insertion. On the basis of in vitro bacteriologic studies, Tatum and co-workers (106) hypothesized that the multifilamental tail of the Dalkon shield may have contributed to the transfer of bacteria from the vagina to the normally sterile uterine cavity. Since then, Sparks and co-workers (102) have implicated the tail of *any* IUD as a possible pathway for bacterial contamination.

Soderstrom (100), using meticulous culture techniques, found that the tails of two of four extrauterine Dalkon Shields contained anaerobic bacterial pathogens; both of these devices were associated with an intraperitoneal inflammatory reaction. The other two Dalkon Shields were found lying free in the abdominal cavity but did not grow pathogenic bacteria.

Although a patient with an extrauterine IUD may be asymptomatic, it is not possible to predict when and if she may become symptomatic or experience complications. It therefore seems reasonable to consider removal of extrauterine IUDs when the diagnosis of perforation is made. The decision to remove an extrauterine IUD requires that the potential complications from the continued presence of the device be weighed against the risks of the potential complications associated with the surgical procedure used to remove it.

Standard surgical procedures for removal of an extrauterine IUD include laparoscopy, laparotomy and colpotomy. None of these operations is free from risk. In experienced hands, laparoscopy appears safer and simpler than either laparotomy or colpotomy. Colpotomy may be used successfully when the IUD is free in the cul-de-sac. If the IUD cannot be located or removed by laparoscopy or colpotomy, laparotomy is required. The cost of hospitalization, days of recovery and the potential morbidity associated with laparotomy are, in general, higher than for either laparoscopy or colpotomy.

At laparoscopy, the location of the IUD can usually be determined without undue difficulty if it is lying free in the pelvic/peritoneal cavity, and it can usually be removed without problems. Laparoscopy has been used for the successful removal of the Lippes Loop, Dalkon Shield, Saf-T-Coil, Margulies Spiral, Birnberg Bow, Cu-T, Cu-7 and Majzlin Spring by numerous investigators (15,27,49,50,54,55,61,72, 74,95,98,100,107,125).

> Soderstrom (100) successfully removed 54 (96.4%) of 56 extrauterine IUDs at laparoscopy. Similar success rates were reported by Zuhair and Buckle (125) who removed 13 (92.9%) of 14 extrauterine IUDs.

IUDs embedded in the omentum or surrounded by adhesions sometimes can be freed laparoscopically by cutting and/or cauterizing the omentum or ad-

hesions. Koetsawang (49) reported on the laparoscopic removal of a Cu-T which was completely covered by adhesions; electrocoagulation was used to
free the device. It should be recognized, however,
that electrocoagulation carries a risk of bowel damage, especially if the adhesions are densely adherent
to the omentum or to the bowel. In the latter situation, it appears to be safer to avoid electrocoagulation and to resort to laparotomy for removal.

Summary

Not all uterine perforations occur at the time of the
IUD insertion, and not all patients with a uterine
perforation have symptoms. The diagnosis of a uterine perforation which occurs at insertion, however,
is often not made until sometime later. This may be
because some of the symptoms associated with a perforated IUD, such as abnormal uterine bleeding or
persistent abdominal cramping, are also experienced
by women with normally placed IUDs in situ and
the possibility of a perforation may not be suspected.
The diagnosis may not be made until the time of a
routine gynecological examination if the strings are
no longer visible and/or pregnancy is suspected.

All types of IUDs are associated with uterine
perforations. The Birnberg Bow is associated with a
significantly higher perforation rate than other IUDs,
but the uterine perforation rates for all other IUDs
are similar. Our review of the literature indicates
that the incidence of uterine perforation with the
Dalkon Shield is probably much lower than the commonly quoted rate of one in 350, and the rate for the
Cu-T is probably higher than the commonly quoted
rate of one in 5,000.

Two factors which appear to be primarily associated with uterine perforations are the IUD insertion
technique and the timing of the insertion. The high-

er rate of uterine perforations with the Birnberg Bow has been attributed to the inserter which ejected the Bow into the uterine cavity. Inadequate training as well as failure to determine the direction and depth of the uterine cavity, failure to diagnosis any cervical or uterine abnormalities or failure to follow the recommended techniques for IUD insertion may increase the risk of uterine perforation.

The design of the IUD does not appear to be directly associated with the incidence of uterine perforation which occurs at the time of insertion. Because the time at which a uterine perforation occurs cannot generally be determined, there is no reliable way to compute the incidence of perforation subsequent to the insertion for different IUDs.

Once the diagnosis of a uterine perforation has been made in an asymptomatic woman, the risks and benefits of IUD removal must be evaluated. The major medical risks of an extrauterine IUD include infection, perforation and strangulation of a portion of bowel. Although these risks are small, they represent major morbidity, and the risks remain present as long as the IUD is located outside the uterus. On the other hand, removal of the extrauterine IUD is not without its own potential risks.

The use of laparoscopy to locate the extrauterine IUD and, if feasible, to remove it may minimize the incidence of complications associated with the surgical removal of IUDs from the abdominal cavity.

References

1. Aitkken, G. W. E., and Verco, C. J. Small bowel perforation by a shield type intrauterine contraceptive device. *Aust. N.Z. J. Obstet. Gynaecol.* 16:187, 1976.

2. Alza Corporation. *The Progestasert.* Intrauterine Progesterone contraceptive system release rated 65 μg/

day for one year. Alza Product Information, Palo Alto, Calif., 1977.

3. Andrews, C. J. Migrating Gräfenberg contraceptive ring. *JAMA* 107:279, 1936.

4. Ansari, A. H. Diagnosis and management of intrauterine device with missing tail. *Obstet. Gynecol.* 44:727, 1974.

5. Athari, T. A., and Pizarro, C. Perforation of the large bowel by a Dalkon Shield intrauterine device. *J. Reprod. Med.* 17:331, 1976.

6. Awon, M. Wandering loops. *J. Obstet. Gynaecol. Brit. Comnwlth.* 73:858, 1966.

7. Badawy, S., and Iskander, S. Omental reaction in cases of uterine perforation by the IUCD. *Contraception* 10:73, 1974.

8. Beasley, W. B. The nurse-midwife as a mediator of contraception. *Am. J. Obstet. Gynecol.* 98:201, 1967.

9. Boria, M. C., and Gordon, M. What to expect when you insert an I.U.D. *Medical Times* 103:98, 1975.

10. Buchman, M. A Study of the intrauterine contraceptive device with and without an extracervical appendage or tail. *Fertil. Steril.* 21:348, 1970.

11. Burnhill, M. S., and Birnberg, C. H. Uterine perforation with intrauterine contraceptive devices. *Acta Obstet. Gynecol.* 98:135, 1967.

12. Cederqvist, L. L.; Lindhe, B-A.; and Fuchs, F. Perforation of the uterus by the Copper-T and Copper-7 intrauterine contraceptive devices. *Acta Obstet. Gynecol.* (Scand) 54:183, 1975.

13. Cederqvist, L. L.; Saary, Z. I.; and Zervoudakis, I. A. Translocation of the Dalkon Shield into the broad ligament. *Obstet. Gynecol.* 46:239, 1975.

14. Chafi, J. Intrauterine contraceptive device. A review and case report of perforation. *J. Maine Med. Assoc.* 62:179, 1971.

15. Cibils, L. A., and Moragne, R. Intra-abdominal Lippes Loop removed at laparoscopy. *J. Reprod. Med.* 6:194, 1971.

16. Cochrane, W. I., and Thomas, M. A. The use of ultrasound B-mode scanning in the localization of intrauterine contraceptive devices. *Radiology* 104:623, 1972.

17. D'Amico, J., and Israel, R. Bowel obstruction and perforation with an intraperitoneal loop intrauterine contraceptive device. *Am. J. Obstet. Gynecol.* 129: 461, 1977.

18. Defoort, P., and Thiery, M. IUD typing by ultrasound —an in vitro study. *Contraception* 9:609, 1974.

19. De Villiers, E. H. Intestinal obstruction following perforation of the uterus with an intra-uterine contraceptive device. *Am. J. Obstet. Gynecol.* 96:592, 1966.

20. Dhall, K.; Dhall, G. I.; and Gupta, B. B. Uterine perforation with the Lippes Loop. *Obstet. Gynecol.* 34: 266, 1969.

21. Diaconis, J. N., and Weiner, C. I. Intrauterine device extraction: a safe method utilizing fluoroscopy. *Radiology* 111:479, 1974.

22. Earley, C. M. Small bowel obstruction due to a Birnberg Bow. *Am. J. Surg.* 113:418, 1967.

23. Echenberg, R., and Ledger, W. J. Peritoneal response to polyethylene foreign bodies. *Obstet. Gynecol.* 31: 795, 1968.

24. Esposito, J. M.; Zarou, D. M.; and Zarou, G. S. Local-

ized inflammation secondary to intraperitoneal IUCD. *J. Reprod. Med.* 8:147, 1972.

25. Eyck, J. V.; Lagasse, A.; and Thiery, M. Scanning electron microscopy of inert and copper-bearing intrauterine devices. *Contraception* 13:65, 1976.

26. Family Planning Research Unit. *Pelvic inflammation, perforation and pregnancy outcome associated with the use of IUDs.* Report no. 15. Exeter: The Family Planning Research Unit, University of Exeter, 1974.

27. Farooqui, M. O., and Shannon, R. H. Removal of Lippes Loop through laparoscopy. *Practitioner* 205: 65, 1970.

28. Friedman, P. J., and Pine, H. L. Radiographic localization of the ectopic intrauterine contraceptive device. *Obstet. Gynecol.* 27:814, 1966.

29. Fuchs, F. F.; Buchman, M. I.; and Nakamoto, M. A new instrument for localization of intrauterine contraceptive devices: the Beolocator. *Am. J. Obstet. Gynecol.* 93:128, 1965.

30. Goldstein, A. I., and Ackerman, E. S. Intrauterine device in the broad ligament. *JAMA* 221:508, 1972.

31. Green, S. C.; Hinkle, D. C.; and Kantor, H. I. Experiences with IUD complications. *Tex. Med.* 66:60, 1970.

32. Guha-Ray, D. K. Translocation of the intrauterine contraceptive device: study of thirty-one cases. *Fertil. Steril.* 28:943, 1977.

33. Gunaratne, M., and Mahroof, H. M. Conversion of a Lippes device into a closed loop: a potential hazard of translocation. *Contraception* 8:357, 1973.

34. Hall, R. E. A reappraisal of intrauterine contraceptive

devices. Prompted by the delayed discovery of uterine perforations. *Am. J. Obstet. Gynecol.* 99:808, 1967.

35. Haspels, A. A. Small bowel obstruction due to perforation by a closed ring type intrauterine device (Antigon). *J. Obstet. Gynecol. Brit. Comnwlth.* 76: 178, 1969.

36. Hasson, H. M. Differential uterine measurements recorded *in vivo. Obstet. Gynecol.* 43:400, 1974.

37. Hefnawi, F.; Hosni, M.; El-Sheikha, Z.; Serour, G. I.; and Hasseeb, F. Perforation of the uterine wall by the Lippes Loop in postpartum women. In *Analysis of intrauterine contraception,* eds. F. Hefnawi and S. J. Segal. New York: American Elsevier Publishing Co., Inc., 1975.

38. Hue, K.; Kwon, H. Y.; Michael, P. H.; and Watson, W. B. A comparative study of the safety and efficacy of postabortal intrauterine contraceptive device insertion. *Am. J. Obstet. Gynecol.* 118:975, 1974.

39. Ianniruberto, A., and Mastroberardino, A. Ultrasonic localization of the Lippes Loop. *Am. J. Obstet. Gynecol.* 114:78, 1972.

40. Janssens, D.; Vrijens, M.; Thiery, M.; and Van Kets, H. Ultrasonic detection, localization and identification of intrauterine contraceptive devices. *Contraception* 8: 485, 1973.

41. Johannisson, E. Recent developments with intrauterine devices. *Contraception* 8:99, 1973.

42. Jones, R. W.; Parker, A.; and Elstein, M. Clinical experience with the Dalkon Shield intrauterine device. *Brit. Med. J.* 3:143, 1973.

43. Jouppila, P. Location of the missing intrauterine contraceptive device. *Acta Obstet. Gynecol.* (Scand) 54: 71, 1975.

44. Kahn, H. S., and Tyler, C. W. Mortality associated with use of IUDs. *JAMA* 234:53, 1975.

45. Kahn, H. S., and Tyler, C. W. An association between the Dalkon Shield and complicated pregnancies among women hospitalized for intrauterine contraceptive device-related disorders. *Am. J. Obstet. Gynecol.* 125:83, 1976.

46. Kamal, I.; Ghoneim, M.; Talaat, M.; and Mallawani, A. The anchoring mechanism of retention of the Copper T device. *Fertil. Steril.* 24:165, 1973.

47. Khatamee, M. A., and Lehfeldt, H. Hysterographic studies in women wearing Copper-T devices. *Adv. Plann. Parent.* X:90, 1975.

48. Kirkpatrick, D.; Schneider, J.; and Peterson, E. P. Large bowel perforation by intrauterine contraceptive devices. *Obstet. Gynecol.* 46:610, 1975.

49. Koetsawang, S. Laparoscopic removal of a perforated Copper-T IUD: a case report. *Contraception* 7:327, 1973.

50. Kozloff, S. R.; Engel, T.; Bernstein, D.; and Silverberg, S. Laparoscopic removal of ectopic intrauterine devices. *Rocky Mt. Med. J.* Nov. 1972.

51. Landesman, R. An intrauterine device extractor. *Obstet. Gynecol.* 37:618, 1971.

52. Lean, T-H. Optimum insertion time for the IUD after delivery. In *Proceedings of the 8th International Conference of IPPF*, April 9–15, Santiago, Chile, 1967.

53. Ledger, W. J., and Willson, J. R. Intrauterine contraceptive devices; the recognition and management of uterine perforations. *Obstet. Gynecol.* 28:806, 1966.

54. Ledward, R. S.; Healey, C.; and Eadie, R. Removal of extrauterine Saf-T-Coil through laparoscopy. *Brit. Med. J.* 1:508, 1972.

55. Leventhal, J. M.; Simon, L. R.; and Shapiro, S. S. Laparoscopic removal of intrauterine contraceptive devices following uterine perforation. *Am. J. Obstet. Gynecol.* 111:102, 1971.

56. Liao, S. C.; Lee, C. H.; and Chow, L. P. Uterine perforation following insertion of the loop. *Am. J. Obstet. Gynecol.* 103:224, 1969.

57. Lippes, J. IUD-related hospitalization and mortality. *JAMA* 235:1001, 1976.

58. Loghmani, M., and Mitra, M. Midwife and doctor insertions of the Copper-T IUD in Isfahan, Iran. Paper presented at the 11th annual meeting of the International Family Planning Research Association, 11–15 Oct. 1975, in Palm Springs, Calif.

59. Marshall, J. Complications of IUDs. In *Contraception today.* Kettering, Northamptonshire: David Green (Printers) Limited, 1971.

60. McArdle, C. R. Ultrasonic localization of missing intrauterine contraceptive devices. *Obstet. Gynecol.* 51: 330, 1978.

61. Merrill, L. K.; Burd, L. I.; and Verburg, D. J. Laparoscopic removal of intraperitoneal Dalkon Shields: a report of three cases. *Am. J. Obstet. Gynecol.* 118: 1146, 1974.

62. Miller, J. F.; Williamson, E.; Morgan, D.; and Elstein, M. A comparison of the Dalkon Shield and Gravigard (Copper 7) intra-uterine devices in Southampton. *Contraception* 13:31, 1976.

63. Mishell, D. R. Current status of contraceptive steroids and the intrauterine device. *Clin. Obstet. Gynecol.* 17:35, 1974.

64. Mosley, W. H.; Chow, L. P.; and Liu, P. T. IUD related hospitalizations. A further analysis of device

specific associations in the 1973 CDC study. Unpublished report from the Department of Population Dynamics. Johns Hopkins University, Baltimore, Maryland, 1974.

65. Murphy, M. C. Migration of a Grafenberg Ring. *Lancet* 2:1369, 1933.

66. Nakamoto, M., and Buchman, M. I. Complications of intrauterine contraceptive devices; report of 5 cases of ectopic placement of the Bow. *Am. J. Obstet. Gynecol.* 94:1073, 1966.

67. Nemes, G., and Kerenyi, T. D. Ultrasonic localization of the IUCD: a new technique. *Am. J. Obstet. Gynecol.* 109:1219, 1971.

68. Neutz, E.; Silber, A.; and Meredino, V. J. Dalkon Shield perforation of the uterus and urinary bladder with calculus formation: case report. *Am. J. Obstet. Gynecol.* 130:848, 1978.

69. Newton, J.; Elias, J.; and Johnson, A. Immediate post-termination insertion of Copper-7 and Dalkon Shield intrauterine contraceptive devices. *J. Obstet. Gynecol. Brit. Comnwlth.* 81:389, 1974.

70. Nygren, K-G., and Johansson, E. D. B. Insertion of the endouterine Copper-T (TCu-200) immediately after first trimester legal abortion. *Contraception* 7:299, 1973.

71. Ostergard, D. R., and Broen, E. M. The insertion of intrauterine devices by physicians and paramedical personnel. *Obstet. Gynecol.* 41:257, 1973.

72. Page, S. W., and Monks, P. L. Laparoscopic removal of an intrauterine device. *Aust. N.Z. J. Obstet. Gynaecol.* 11:192, 1971.

73. Pastene, L.; Rivera, M.; Zipper, J.; Medel, M.; and Thomas, M. IUD insertions by midwives: five years

experience in Santiago, Chile. *Int. J. Gynaecol. Obstet.* 15:84, 1977.

74. Pearce, D. J. Laparoscopic removal of IUDs from the abdomen. *Brit. Med. J.* 1:1017, 1976.

75. Piiroinen, O. Ultrasonic localization of intrauterine contraceptive devices. *Acta Obstet. Gynecol.* (Scand) 51:203, 1972.

76. Price, C. W. R. An unusual cause of intestinal obstruction. *Med. J. Australia.* January 22, 1955.

77. Post, D. F. Perforation of the uterus and partial extrusion of a Lippes Loop. *Obstet. Gynecol.* 34:859, 1969.

78. Quakernack, K.; Schmidt, E. H.; Lieder, B.; and Beller, F. K. The identification of IUD by ultrasound in the uterine cavity. *Eur. J. Obstet. Gynecol. Reprod. Biol.* 4:203, 1975.

79. Ratnam, S. S., and Tow, S. H. Translocation of the loop. In *Post partum family planning. A report on the international program*, ed., G. I. Zatuchni. New York: McGraw-Hill Book Co., 1970.

80. Ratnam, S. S., and Yin, J. C. K. Translocation of Lippes Loop (the missing Loop). *Brit. Med. J.* 1:612, 1968.

81. Rimdusit, S., and Mishell, D. R. Determining the location of intrauterine devices with the Beolocator. *Obstet. Gynecol.* 31:132, 1968.

82. Roberts, J. M., and Ledger, W. J. Operative removal of intraperitoneal intrauterine contraceptive devices —a reappraisal. *Am. J. Obstet. Gynecol.* 112:863, 1972.

83. Rubin, A. Complications due to Lippes Loop: report of a death and other complications seen over an 18-

month period at Baragwanath Hospital. *S. Afr. J. Obstet. Gynaecol.* 10:45, 1972.

84. Rutherford, A. M. The Grafenberg Ring. *N.Z. Med. J.* 60:413, 1961.

85. Saronwala, K. C.; Singh, R.; and Dass, H. Lippes Loop perforation of the uterus and urinary bladder with stone formation. *Obstet. Gynecol.* 44:424, 1974.

86. Schwartz, G. F., and Markowitz, A. M. Richter's hernia resulting from displaced intrauterine contraceptive device. *Am. Surg.* Aug. 1970, p. 502.

87. Schwartz, G. F., and Markowitz, A. M. Serious sequelae of intrauterine contraceptive devices. *JAMA* 211:959, 1970.

88. Scott, R. B. Critical illnesses and deaths associated with intrauterine devices. *Obstet. Gynecol.* 31:322, 1968.

89. Scutchfield, F. D., and Long, W. N. Perforation of the uterus with the Lippes Loop. *JAMA* 208:2335, 1969.

90. Segal, S. J., and Atkinson, L. E. In Changing concepts of intrauterine contraception. *Progress in Gynecology*, V. VI., eds. M. L. Taymor and T. H. Green. New York: Grune & Stratton, 1975.

91. Segal, S. J., and Tietze, C. Contraceptive technology: current and prospective methods. In *Reports on population/family planning, the Population Council.* New York: Columbia University Press, 1969.

92. Seward, P. J.; Burns, G. T.; and Quattlebaum, E. G. Intra-uterine contraception. An unusual complication. *JAMA* 194:1385, 1965.

93. Shapiro, A. G. Management of the lost intrauterine contraceptive device. *Obstet. Gynecol.* 49:238, 1977.

94. Shimkin, P. M.; Siegel, H. A.; and Seaman, W. B. Radiographic aspects of perforated intrauterine contraceptive devices. *Radiology* 92:353, 1969.

95. Siegler, A. M. Removal of ectopic intrauterine contraceptive devices aided by laparoscopy. *Am. J. Obstet. Gynecol.* 115:158, 1973.

96. Siegler, A. M., and Kemmann, E. Hysteroscopic removal of occult intrauterine contraceptive device. *Obstet. Gynecol.* 46:604, 1975.

97. Slaughter, L., and Morris, D. J. Peritoneal-cutaneous fistula secondary to a perforated Dalkon Shield. *Am. J. Obstet. Gynecol.* 124:206, 1976.

98. Smith, D. C. Removal of an ectopic IUD through the laparoscope. *Am. J. Obstet. Gynecol.* 105:285, 1969.

99. Snowden, R., and Williams, M. The use-effectiveness of the Dalkon Shield in the United Kingdom. *Contraception* 7:91, 1972.

100. Soderstrom, R. M. The wandering IUD—what to do? In *Risks, benefits, and controversies in fertility control*, eds. J. J. Sciarra, G. I. Zatuchni and J. J. Speidel. Maryland: Harper & Row, 1978.

101. Somboonsuk, A.; Khaopurisuthi, V.; Boonsiri, B.; and Reinprayoon, D. IUD perforation: 11 years experience. In *Proceedings, The Seventh Asian Congress of Obstetrics and Gynecology*, Bangkok, Thailand, 1977, pp. 460–466.

102. Sparks, R. A.; Purrier, B. G. A.; Watt, P. J.; and Elstein, M. The bacteriology of the cervical canal in relation to the use of an intrauterine contraceptive device. Paper presented at The Uterine Cervix in Reproduction Workshop Conference, 24–26 June, 1977, Rottach-Eqern, West Germany.

103. Sprague, A. D., and Jenkins, V. R. Perforation of the

uterus with a shield intrauterine device. *Obstet. Gynecol.* 41:80, 1973.

104. Tatum, H. J. Contraception with the endouterine Copper T: a preliminary report. *Adv. Plann. Parent.* VII:92, 1972.

105. Tatum, H. J. Metallic copper as an intrauterine contraceptive agent. *Am. J. Obstet. Gynecol.* 117: 602, 1973.

106. Tatum, H. J.; Schmidt, F. H.; Phillips, D.; McCarty, M.; and O'Leary, W. M. The Dalkon Shield contro-versy: structural and bacteriological studies of IUD tails. *JAMA* 231:711, 1975.

107. Taylor, M. B., and White, M. F. Operative laparo-scopy: removal of intra-abdominal IUD with biopsy tongs. *Obstet. Gynecol.* 35:981, 1970.

108. Thambu, J. Complication following insertion of in-trauterine contraceptive device. *Brit. Med. J.* 2:407, 1965.

109. Thomsen, R. P. IUD complications—radiological aspects of diagnosis. *Comtemp. Obstet. Gynecol.* 5: 77, 1975.

110. Tietze, C. Contraception with intrauterine devices 1959—1966. *Am. J. Obstet. Gynecol.* 96:1043, 1966.

111. Timonen, H., and Luukkainen, T. Immediate post-abortion insertion of the Copper T (TCu 200) with 18 months follow up. *Contraception* 9:153, 1974.

112. Toppozada, H. K.; Rizk, M. A.; Khowessah, M. M.; Loutfi, I.; Hamdi, A.; and El Deeb, A. Radiologic aids to localization of an extrauterine intrauterine contra-ceptive device. *Fertil. Steril.* 24:170, 1973.

113. Totterman, L. E., and Karjalainen, K-L. Localization of a missing IUD with the help of plain x-ray exami-

nation and a second IUD. *Acta Obstet. Gynecol.* (Scand) 49:139, 1970.

114. Tsai, W-S.; Chen, H-Y.; Chen, Y-P.; and Wei, P-Y. The uterus and a consideration of a causative factor of accidental pregnancy. *Int. J. Fertil.* 18:85, 1973.

115. Tushuizen, P. B. Th., and Ubacks, J. M. H. Perforation of the large bowel by a Lippes Loop. *J. Obstet. Gynaecol. Brit. Comnwlth.* 89:854, 1973.

116. Valle, R. F., and Freeman, D. W. Hysteroscopy in the localization and removal of intrauterine devices with "missing strings." *Contraception* 11:161, 1975.

117. Valle, R. F., and Freeman, D. W. Hysteroscopy in the management of the "lost" intrauterine device. *Adv. Plann. Parent.* X:164, 1975.

118. Valle, R. F.; Sciarra, J.; and Freeman, D. W. Hysteroscopic removal of intrauterine devices with missing filaments. *Obstet. Gynecol.* 49:55, 1977.

119. Wei, P-Y. Perforation of the uterine wall by the Lippes Loop. Its frequency and mechanism. *Am. J. Obstet. Gynecol.* 101:770, 1968.

120. Whitson, L. G.; Israel, R.; and Bernstein, G. S. The extrauterine Dalkon Shield. *Obstet. Gynecol.* 44:418, 1974.

121. Wiknjosastro, H.; Doodoh, A.; Rachman, I.; Agussjaries, Harap H.; Mitra, M.; and Thomas, M. Postpartum use of the Lippes Loop and Dalkon Shield. In *Proceedings of 1st Inter-Congress*, ed. S. M. M. Karim, Singapore, 1976.

122. Williamson, H. O.; Bank, H. L.; and Kirkland, B. H.; Tatum, T.: experience with 3000 patients. *Adv. Plann. Parent.* X:95, 1975.

123. Winters, H. S. Ultrasound detection of intrauterine

contraceptive devices. *Am. J. Obstet. Gynecol.* 95: 880, 1966.

124. Wittmann, B. K., and Chow, T. T. S. Diagnostic ultrasound in the management of patients using intrauterine contraceptive devices. *Brit. J. Obstet. Gynaecol.* 83:802, 1976.

125. Zuhair, A., and Buckle, A. E. R. Uterine perforation by intrauterine contraceptive devices and their laparoscopic removal. *Int. J. Gynaecol. Obstet.* 13:101, 1975.

Chapter 4

Pelvic inflammatory disease

Introduction

In 1937, a letter to the Editor of the Journal of the American Medical Association inquired about the safety of intrauterine silver rings. The Editor's reply listed several case reports of severe pelvic infection and death among users of intrauterine devices (3). During the next two decades, additional case reports of infectious complications of IUDs occasionally appeared. It was not, however, until the 1960s and 1970s that epidemiologic studies were undertaken to assess any association between the use of IUDs and pelvic inflammatory disease (PID).

The first major IUD study which reported on PID rates among users of different IUDs was that of the Cooperative Statistical Program (CSP) for the Evaluation of Intrauterine Devices. The study included 23,917 first insertions of different nonmedicated IUDs. In the final report of the CSP (95), no significant differences were reported in PID rates for women using different types of IUDs. The two-year cumulative life table rates of PID per 100 women were 3.8 for Lippes Loops, 3.6 for Margulies Spirals, 4.2 for Birnberg Bows, 4.1 for steel rings and 5.2 for the Saf-T-Coil. Similar data were not collected among a comparable group of women who did not use IUDs. The CSP report, therefore, did not assess whether the risk of acquiring a pelvic infection was increased

for women who used intrauterine contraceptive
devices.

Since the publication of the CSP report, a number of investigations have been conducted specifically to assess the risk of PID among IUD users compared to women who do not use IUDs. Other investigators who have studied and evaluated specific IUDs
have reported on the occurrence of PID among users
of these devices. The literature also includes reports
of isolated cases of PID without reference to any
known population of IUD users or nonusers.

This chapter summarizes the results of many
reports based on different definitions of PID and
varying study methodologies. Only the association
between IUD use and pelvic infection among non-
pregnant women will be considered. Discussion of
the association between IUD use and pelvic infection in pregnant women is considered in Chapter 7.

Definitions

"Pelvic inflammatory disease" (PID) is a general
term which refers to an inflammatory condition of
the upper female genital tract. Clinically, the term
PID is most often used to denote either an acute or
chronic infectious condition of the fallopian tubes
and/or the sequelae of such infections, such as tubo-
ovarian adhesions, hydrosalpinx or tubo-ovarian
abscess. The criteria for the diagnosis of PID vary
considerably. To represent accurately the data reported in the literature, we have not edited or
changed the authors' definitions of PID or imposed a
uniform definition of PID.

Studies which present data regarding a possible
association between IUD use and PID fall into one or
more of the following categories: 1) bacteriologic,
2) histopathologic, 3) epidemiologic or 4) clinical,
including case reports.

Bacteriologic Studies

To assess the possible effects of IUDs in the etiology of pelvic infection, several investigators have studied changes in the bacterial flora of the endometrial cavity subsequent to IUD insertion.

In a study of 200 women, Willson and co-workers (100) obtained cervical and endometrial secretions for culture prior to insertion of a Margulies spiral and again after insertion at intervals up to a maximum period of 24 months. No significant alteration in the flora of the endometrial cavity was found after IUD insertion. Sixteen (8%) patients developed infections, but only four were considered to be due to the presence of the IUD.

Sen and co-workers (82) examined material obtained by cervical swab for the presence of bacteria and fungi before and after the insertion of Lippes Loops in 787 women. No significant difference in the percentage of positive cultures was found, and no clinically recognizable pelvic infections were reported.

Golditch and Huston (30) evaluated endometrial cultures from 117 women who had used an IUD (unspecified device) for six or more months and from 104 women who used no IUD. The proportions of positive cultures were similar in both groups. Most of the organisms that grew on culture were normal to the vaginal flora, but anaerobic organisms were recovered from a significantly higher proportion of the IUD users than from the nonusers.

Salmi and co-workers (77) evaluated the cervical bacterial flora of 60 women who had Cu-Ts and 25 who had Lippes Loops inserted. Although the bacterial flora was increased slightly in diversity and amount at three and six months after IUD insertion, there were no differences in the cervical bacterial flora between the users of the two IUDs.

To avoid the problem of contaminating the endometrial cultures by endocervical or vaginal organisms, Mishell and co-workers (63) obtained transfundal aerobic and anaerobic cultures of the endometrial cavity from the uteri of 61 patients who had IUDs inserted at varying times before hysterectomy. The cultures were positive in all cases when the IUD had been inserted 24 hours or less before surgery. There were no positive cultures if the IUDs were inserted 30 days or more before surgery. The authors concluded that the insertion of an IUD results in contamination of the endometrial cavity with bacteria from the vagina or cervix, but that such bacteria are cleared from the uterine cavity within a short period of time.

In addition to the concern that bacteria from the lower genital tract may contaminate the upper genital tract, attention has focused specifically on the possible influence of IUDs on gonorrheal infections. In the past, many clinicians were of the opinion that the majority of patients with acute salpingitis had gonococcal infections of the fallopian tubes. Study of more recent data, however, requires modification of this opinion.

Hager and Wiesner (35) reviewed the epidemiology of acute salpingitis. They found that only 10% to 17% of women with culture proven gonorrhea developed PID, and that the proportion of women with salpingitis caused by gonococcal infections varied from 30% to 80%.

Statham and Morton (88) suggested that the morbidity of gonorrhea is increased by the presence of an IUD (unspecified devices). They based their contention on their observations of three women (42.9%) with PID out of seven IUD users who had gonorrhea. This rate is similar to the 20% to 40% risk of acute salpingitis which occurred among women who do not use IUDs and who are exposed to N. gonorrhea (51).

In a review of the etiology of acute PID, Eschenbach and Holmes (23) reported that N. gonorrhea was isolated from the endocervix in 33% to 51% of women with acute PID. The presence of N. gonorrhea in the cervix, however, does not necessarily prove that it is present in the upper genital tract or that it is the causative agent of the upper genital infection.

Lip and Burgoyne (53), in an evaluation of 49 patients with acute salpingitis, found 38.9% of the cul-de-sac cultures positive for N. gonorrhea compared to 46.9% of the cervical cultures.

In contrast, Mardh and Westrom (57) cultured N. gonorrhea from the lower genital tract in 34% of 50 women with acute salpingitis, but none of the cul-de-sac cultures was positive for N. gonorrhea.

Chow and co-workers (11) commented that the high frequency of positive cultures for N. gonorrhea from the lower genital tract and the infrequent occurrence of positive cultures for N. gonorrhea from the fallopian tubes, adnexae or cul-de-sac suggests that the gonococcus may pave the way for secondary invaders from the normal vaginal flora to gain access to the upper genital tract. Chow and co-workers (11) cultured specimens obtained by culdocentesis and identified gonococci in only one of 20 patients in spite of positive cervical cultures for N. gonorrhea in 13 (65%) of these patients. Cultures of cul-de-sac aspirates were positive for a variety of aerobic and anaerobic organisms in 18 of the 20 patients.

The possible role of the cervicovaginal appendage or "tail" of the IUD in the development of upper genital tract infections is not completely understood.

Mishell and co-workers (63) obtained transfundal cultures of the endometrial cavities of 61 women who underwent hysterectomy three hours to seven months after insertion of Lippes Loops. Their data do not implicate the tail of the IUD in promoting bacterial ascent from the lower to the upper genital tract.

Willson and co-workers (102) found no significant differences in the incidence of upper genital tract infections or infections localized to the cervix between the Margulies Spiral with a tail (7.0%, 0.9%) and the same IUD without a tail (5.5%, 0.5%).

Buchman (9) found no significant differences in endocervical bacteriologic cultures obtained from women using Birnberg Bows or Lippes Loops with or without tails. The incidence of PID was similar for bows with or without tails (3.9% versus 3.0%) and for loops with or without tails (0.9% versus 0.5%).

Burnhill (10) found no difference in the frequency and distribution of positive cultures from IUDs with tails (50 bows, 1 loop, 1 spiral, 1 spring) and from those without tails (80 bows).

Tietze and Lewit (95) reported no significant differences between the overall PID rates or removal rates for PID associated with IUDs with tails (loops, spirals, coils) and those without tails (rings and bows).

In contrast to these studies, Elstein (21) reported an 18.1% rate of pelvic infection among 149 users of Lippes Loops with tails compared to 0.8% for 128 users of Birnberg Bows without tails.

Bacteriologic in vitro studies of IUD tails from removed Dalkon Shields have suggested that a multifilamental IUD tail may contribute to the transfer of bacteria from the vagina to the normally sterile uterine cavity (91).

Sparks and co-workers (84) have suggested that the presence of any kind of tail may interfere with the protective mechanisms of the cervix and permit bacteria to ascend from the vagina to the uterine cavity along the outside of the tail of the IUD. The bacteriology of the uterus and cervix from hysterectomy specimens which contained Dalkon Shields without tails was found to be similar to the bacteriology of hysterectomy specimens from 50 women who did not use IUDs. On the other hand, the bacteriology of 11 hysterectomy specimens which contained nine IUDs with multifilament tails and two IUDs with monofilament tails was similar to that of the vagina, thus implicating the IUD tail in the ascent of bacteria from the vagina.

It is apparent from these varying reports that further clinical and bacteriologic studies will be required to delineate the precise role of the IUD and its tail in the pathogenesis of pelvic inflammatory disease.

Since Hagenfeldt's (34) demonstration that the concentration of copper is significantly increased in the endometrial secretions and cervical mucus of women who use copper-bearing IUDs, some authors have suggested that use of such devices may be protective against gonococcal infections.

From the results of *in vitro* studies, Fiscina and co-workers (26) and Spence and co-workers (87) inferred that micromolar amounts of copper may inhibit the growth of *N. gonorrhea*.

Cohen and Thomas (13) reported three cases of women who were using copper-bearing IUDs and who did not contract gonorrhea after vaginal intercourse with men who had documented urethral gonorrhea.

Other studies, however, have found no evidence that copper-bearing IUDs (Cu-7-200 and Cu-T-200) have a protective effect against gonorrheal infections.

Among 93 women who were using a Cu-T-200, positive cultures for *N. gonorrhea* were obtained from 7.5%. Only 1.1% of the women had clinically diagnosed pelvic infections. The corresponding rates for 62 women who were using Dalkon Shields were

8.1% and 3.2%. The rates for the two IUDs were not significantly different (85).

Among 97 women who were using either Cu-7-200 devices or Cu-T-200 devices and who had laparoscopically verified diagnoses of salpingitis, 13.4% had positive cultures for N. *gonorrhea*; the corresponding rate among 28 women using Lippes Loops or Saf-T-Coils was 14.3% (98).

The available evidence suggests that the prevalence rates of gonorrhea are similar for IUD users and for oral contraceptive users.

Johannisson and co-workers (42) found similar infection rates of gonorrhea for women using copper-bearing IUDs and for women using oral contraceptives. Berger and co-workers (7) reported the prevalence of asymptomatic cervical gonorrhea among oral contraceptive users to be 10.6%, compared to 9.5% for IUD users (unspecified device) and 1.7% for users of condoms, diaphragms or foams. However, McCormack and co-workers (60) found among women with gonococcal infections that the proportions of women with anogenital gonorrhea who were either asymptomatic or had nonspecific symptoms significantly differed by the type of contraceptive practice: no method of contraception, 41.3%; oral contraception, 58.6%, IUD, 14.3%; other methods, 60.0%.

From these studies there is no evidence that the IUD protects against gonorrheal infections, but it is unclear whether it facilitates the rate of development of clinical PID in women with asymptomatic gonorrhea. Any study of the possible effect of the IUD on gonococcal infection must recognize that the incidence of PID among IUD users is related to the prevalence of gonorrhea in the community. In communities where gonorrhea is common, high rates of PID among IUD users can be anticipated, regardless of the types of IUDs used. One of the shortcomings of many studies is that the number and/or proportion of gonorrhea-related infections in the reference population is not stated.

Histopathologic Studies

Chronic endometritis, defined histopathologically by the presence of plasma cells and lymphocytes, often with histiocyte infiltration, stromal edema, vascular congestion and occasional fibroblast proliferation, is generally present among women who use IUDs. It is usually limited to the endometrium in the immediate vicinity of the IUD. The presence of this inflammatory response is thought by some to be essential to the antifertility effects of the IUD (63,66). Evidence of chronic endometritis, however, can not always be documented in all IUD users.

There is evidence of an increased prevalence of chronic endometritis among IUD users who are asymptomatic.

> Willson and co-workers (101) found no bacteriologic differences in cultures taken before insertion of a Margulies Spiral IUD and those taken after several months of IUD use among women who had neither abnormal bleeding nor other pelvic symptoms. However, 14 of 27 endometrial biopsies obtained from women with abnormal bleeding and/or complaints showed evidence of endometritis.
>
> Lippes (54) reported that endometritis was diagnosed in 4.7% of the endometrial biopsies from 150 asymptomatic Lippes Loop users who had used the IUD for six or more months, and from 1.3% of the endometrial biopsies in women who had not used the Loop. Among the IUD users, the endometritis was considered a "sterile endometritis" or "foreign body reaction."
>
> Israel and Davis (40) evaluated hysterectomy specimens from 46 women who had used an IUD (a

closed plastic ring or shield device) for 1.5 to 8.0 months and from 46 women who had not used an IUD. A pathologic diagnosis of chronic endometritis was made in 13.0% of the IUD users and in 2.2% of the nonusers.

Lee and co-workers (52) obtained endometrial biopsies from 422 IUD (Lippes Loop and Margulies Spiral) users. The overall incidence of abnormal endometrial changes was 9.2%. There were only 8 (1.9%) cases of chronic endometritis. Most women (81.7%) had used the IUD for less than one year.

Ober and co-workers (70) evaluated endometrial biopsy specimens from 93 asymptomatic IUD users (Lippes Loops, Margulies Spirals, Birnberg Bows) and 107 symptomatic IUD users (women who had their IUDs removed because of abnormal or excessive bleeding, pelvic pain, persistent vaginal discharge and other symptoms). The study included women who had used an IUD for up to 105 months. For the asymptomatic women, 9.7% of the biopsies showed inflammatory changes, compared to 25.2% of the biopsies for the symptomatic women.

Ober and co-workers (68) reported endometritis in 78.6% of the endometrial biopsies from 56 women who had symptoms (abnormal bleeding, discharge or pain) requiring removal of their Majzlin Springs, compared to 16.6% of the endometrial biopsies from 12 asymptomatic women.

Ober and co-workers (69), in an evaluation of 393 women, reported biopsy evidence of endometritis in 2.5% of the 266 asymptomatic women who had used Lippes Loops for 36 months or more, compared to 21.2% of the 52 asymptomatic women who had used Lippes Loops for 18–35 months and 44.4% of the 54 women who had used Lippes Loops for 36 months or more.

Kulka and co-workers (50) reported endometritis in 84.6% of the endometrial biopsies from 13 IUD users who complained of abnormal bleeding, pain or severe discharge and who hadheir IUDs (Majzlin Springs) removed.

Philips and co-workers (74) reported that endometrial biopsies were indicative of endometritis in 17.2% of 132 women who had used a Lippes Loop for 3 to 5 years and in 25.0% of women who had used a Lippes Loop for 5 to 9 years.

These studies confirm that changes in endometrial histopathology do occur in association with IUD use. Various investigators have reported a wide range of rates of chronic endometritis among asymptomatic and symptomatic IUD users. These findings highlight the types of problems which occur in studies regarding the diagnosis of PID and the reasons for discontinuation of IUD use. For example, many women with IUD-related symptoms (e.g., abnormal uterine bleeding and/or pain) may have pelvic infections, but a clinical diagnosis of pelvic infection may not be made when their IUDs are removed. In such cases, the removal may be categorized as a removal for pain and/or bleeding, rather than a removal for PID.

Epidemiologic Studies

In 1977, the FDA's Panel on Review of Obstetrical-Gynecological Devices recommended that IUD package labeling include the statement that "IUD use is associated with a 3- to 5-fold increase in infection rate" (4). The FDA recommendation was based largely on the results of several epidemiologic studies.

Table 4.1 presents pertinent information on studies designed to assess the relationship between PID and IUD use. The first six reports listed in the table are all case-control studies in which the prevalence of IUD use among a group of women with PID (cases) is compared to a group of women without

Table 4.1 Summary of studies to assess the association of pelvic inflammatory disease and IUD use.

Reference Number	Study Description	Odds Ratio (95% Confidence Limits)	Results/Comments
90	Case-control. 50 emergency room patients with a putative diagnosis of PID. 50 controls no. 1: women attending general medical clinic. 50 controls no. 2: women appearing with sick children in pediatric emergency room. Cases matched to controls by age, marital status and time since last pregnancy.	9.3 (4.2–20.9)	PID diagnostic criteria: Temperature 99.8F and above, and 2 of the following: lower abdominal pain and tenderness, cervical motion tenderness, adnexal tenderness. The control groups were similar with respect to their contraceptive practice distributions. Types of IUDs not stated.
55	Case-control. 91 cases with a hospital discharge diagnosis of PID, salpingitis, endometritis. 38 controls discharged from same hospital with admitting diagnosis of acute appendicitis.	1.9 (0.5–7.2)	Types of IUDs not stated.
24	Case-control. 50 febrile cases (temperature of ≥ 38C), 100 afebrile cases, 100 controls. Cases: uterine or adnexal tenderness on pelvic examination, no diagnosis other than PID to explain "illness" at initial emergency room visit or within 1 month. Controls: emergency room patients without complaint of abdominal pain or discomfort, and without diagnosis of any gynecologic problem.	5.1 (2.5–10.5) for febrile cases. 2.7 (1.4–5.0) for afebrile cases.	Past diagnosis of PID: febrile cases, 58%; afebrile cases, 75%; controls, 43.5%. IUDs: Lippes Loop, Saf-T-Coil, Dalkon Shield, Cu-7.

98	Case-control. 515 cases of laparoscopically verified acute salpingitis. 1,545 controls: women matched for age and date of birth selected from a regional population register, contacted by a postal questionnaire (response rate 78.8%). 156 controls excluded for a number of reasons (e.g., current pregnancy). Excluded women using no contraception. Only 741 controls included in analysis.	3.0 (2.2–4.1)	IUDs: Lippes Loop, Saf-T-Coil, Cu-T, Cu-7

| 32 | Reanalysis of data from Westrom and co-workers (98). |

Age	Multips	Nullips
16–20	1.1	8.1*
21–25	1.1	7.5*
26–30	1.6	2.6
31–35	3.1	—

* Significantly different from 1 (p < 0.10)

Only nulliparous women ≤ 25 years of age at an increased risk of PID.

| 22 | Case-control. 173 cases; 173 controls matched for age, race, marital status, parity, number of sex partners, presence of gonorrhea. | 4.4 (1.9–5.7) | Odds ratio = 2.8 for gonococcal PID; 6.5 for nongonococcal PID. IUDs: Dalkon Shield, Lippes Loop, Saf-T-Coil, Cu-7. |

Table 4.1 (cont'd)

Reference Number	Study Description	Odds Ratio (95% Confidence Limits)	Results/Comments
94	Case-control. 101 cases, women with recurrent PID were excluded. 101 controls matched for age, current marital status, interval since last pregnancy termination.	3.3 (0.9–5.9)	Types of IUDs not stated.
106	Incidence of acute PID documented in a poor urban population in a 1 year period. 902 acute first episodes of PID; 478 termed definite.		PID diagnostic criteria: Temperature over 99.8F, lower abdominal cervical motion tenderness, visualization of acute supracervical pelvic inflammation at laparotomy. Attack rates/1,000 woman-years of first definite episode of PID among women within one year of pregnancy termination: IUD—66.2 Oral—13.4 Vaginal foam—25.2 Attack rate for overall female population (15–44 years of age) 9.6/1,000 women per year.

67	Gonorrhea screening program. 1,706 women screened over a 9-month period. Symptoms of PID: complaints of pelvic pain or abdominal cramping other than during menstruation or pelvic tenderness on physical examination.	2.2 (1.8–2.7) for women with symptoms of PID.	Method	Percentage with Symptoms

Method	Percentage with Symptoms
Oral	20.6
IUD	33.3
Other	16.2

Method	Percentage with Gonococcal PID
Oral	0.7
IUD	3.1
Other	0.2

15	1,583 consecutive cases of sterilization at 4 hospitals. Evidence of PID noted by surgeons.	Evidence of PID: tubal adhesions, hydrosalpinx, adnexitis, uterine adhesions, enlarged ovary.

Contraceptive Method	Percentage of Cases with Tubal Adhesions
Never used (N = 213)	8.9
IUD only (N = 162)	12.3
Pill only (N = 612)	4.9

Rates for never used and IUD-only group not different ($p > .10$). Pill-only rates lower than rates for never used and IUD-only groups ($p < .05$).

Table 4.1 (cont'd)

Reference Number	Study Description	Odds Ratio (95% Confidence Limits)	Results/Comments
73	Observations of PID in 200 women undergoing transvaginal tubal sterilization. Retrospective study based on operative notes.	12.3 (4.4–34.0)	Criteria for diagnosing PID included 1 or more of the following: adhesions, congestion, tubal occlusion with clubbing, oozing of pus from fimbria.

Contraceptive PID

Method	Number	Percentage
IUD (N = 101)	28	27.7
Hormonal (N = 73)	3	4.1
None (N = 26)	0	0.0

Risk of PID increased with duration of IUD use:

Time from IUD Insertion

Years	Percentage of Cases with PID
<1	13
1–3	24
4–6	28
76+	50

| 83 | Histologic examination of tubal specimens from 49 IUD users and from 1,500 nonusers. All patients underwent voluntary laparoscopic sterilization. | Nonbacterial chronic salpingitis noted in 46.9% of IUD users versus 0.7% of nonusers. Among the IUD users, those with normal oviducts or salpingitus were similar in terms of age, race, marital status, parity, type of IUD, duration of IUD use and symptoms. IUD types: Dalkon Shield, Lippes Loop, Saf-T-Coil, Majzlin Spring; 44.9% were Dalkon Shields and reflected use of the Shield in the community. |

| 96 | Long-term follow-up study of 17,032 white women aged 25–39 using different methods of contraception in 17 family planning clinics. Prospective study. | 1st event rates/1,000 woman years of salpingitis, PID, endometritis standardized for age, parity, social class, smoking |

	IUD user	Nonuser
In-patient only	2.02	0.57
In-patient and Out-patient	2.59	0.94

IUD user rates significantly higher than nonuser rates (p < 0.01)

PID (controls). For each case-control study the computed odds ratio and its 95% confidence limits are given. The odds ratio, sometimes referred to as the "relative risk," is the ratio of the odds that an IUD user will have PID to the odds that a nonuser will have PID. The odds ratio is not the same as relative risk, which is the ratio of the probability of PID among IUD users to the probability of PID among nonusers. Relative risk can be computed directly only in cohort studies. Under certain circumstances, the odds ratio can be used to approximate the relative risk. In Appendix B, a more detailed discussion of the odds ratio and relative risk is given. When the odds ratios and their approximate 95% confidence limits presented in Table 4.1 were not provided by the investigators, they were computed by the authors according to the methods of Fleiss (27) and Miettinen (62), respectively.

In each of the six case-control studies, a higher proportion of women with PID (cases) were IUD users than were those without PID (controls). The computed odds ratios from four of these studies (22, 24,90,98) are significantly greater than one, implying an increased risk of PID among IUD users than for nonusers. The odds ratio in these four studies are significantly different from each other (p<.05; based on the Mantel-Haenzel procedure), so that a pooled odds ratio for the four studies has not been computed. Nevertheless, it appears that the odds of an IUD user having acute PID is higher than that of a nonuser, and that the apparent increased risk of PID cannot be attributed to any specific IUD type or configuration.

Gray (32), in a reanalysis of the data from the case-control study of Westrom and co-workers (98), found that when women were grouped into various age categories the odds ratio was significantly greater than one only for nulliparous women under the age of 26. Other epidemiologic studies have not reported a higher risk of PID for nulliparous women.

Table 4.2 *Estimated PID rates (per 1,000 women per year) among IUD users and nonusers.*

Assumed PID Rate in General Population	Estimated PID Rate		
	IUD Users	Nonusers	Difference in Rates for Users and Nonusers
1	2.0	0.9	1.1
5	9.8	4.4	5.4
10	19.4	8.7	10.7
15	29.0	13.1	15.9
20	38.5	17.5	21.0
25	47.9	21.8	26.1
30	57.2	26.2	31.0

Moreover, clinical studies reported in the literature have not found a higher incidence of PID among nulliparous compared to multiparous women.

Osser and co-workers (71) reported a study of 750 women who had Cu-T IUDs inserted and were followed up for one year. The percentages of nulliparous and parous women who had a laparoscopically confirmed diagnosis of PID were 3.8% and 1.5%, respectively. The differences between these rates were not found to be statistically significant. Also, among the women in the high-risk age group (16 to 25), the PID rates were 4.7% and 4.2% for nulliparas and Multiparas.

From the data presented in the case-control studies, estimates of the proportions of IUD users and nonusers who have PID can be obtained by assuming various proportions of women in the general population who have PID (16). Such estimates are shown in Table 4.2. This table shows an increased risk of PID attributable to IUD use of 1.1 per 1,000 women per year if the PID rate in the general population is assumed to be 1.0 per 1,000 women per year. The attributable risk increases to 31.0 per 1,000 women per year if the PID rate in the general population is assumed to be 30 per 1,000 women per year. Assuming the annual incidence of PID is 1.36%

among women of reproductive age (the rate reported by Eschenbach [22], for women aged 14–34 in the United States), the increased risk of PID attributable to IUD use is estimated to be 14.5 per 1,000 women per year. Such estimates are valid only if it can be assumed that the PID (cases) and no PID (control) groups in the case-control studies are representative of these same groups in the general population. This assumption may be challenged, however, on the basis that the case-control studies reported in Table 4.1 involve only women seen in hospitals and do not include cases of PID treated in other than hospital settings.

Although the odds ratio is a useful measure of association in case-control studies, this statistic does not provide an estimate of the magnitude of the risk of acquiring PID among either the groups of IUD users or nonusers. Furthermore, a statistically significant odds ratio may be obtained by either an over-representation of IUD users in the PID group or by an under-representation of IUD users in the control group. For example, there is some evidence that women who use oral contraceptives may be at a reduced risk of PID compared to women who do not use oral contraceptives (15,22,24,106). Thus, their inclusion in any control group might be expected to increase the odds ratios reported in the case-control studies. Reanalysis of the Faulkner and Ory (24) data gives significantly higher odds ratios for those who do not use oral contraceptives than for those who use oral contraceptives. In the febrile and in the afebrile groups, these odds ratios were 2.5 and 2.1, respectively. Both of these ratios were significantly (p<.05) greater than one, and indicate an increased risk of PID for women who do not use oral contraceptives than for women who do use them. Also, in the study by Eschenbach and co-workers (22) the odds ratio (2.0) was significantly greater than one (p<.05) for nonusers of oral contraceptives compared to users. Thus, if use of oral contraceptives is associated with reduced rates of PID, then the inclusion of different proportions of oral contraceptive users of the case and control groups might seriously bias the results of these studies.

Although the case-control studies have shown an association between IUD use and PID, the following limitations to these studies should be recognized.

1. The control group should be selected with attention to appropriate detail. If one or more control subjects are matched to each case, then the matching should be with respect to relevant criteria. The difficulty in defining an appropriate control group can be seen from the studies in Table 4.1. The control groups included emergency room patients without gynecological problems, patients admitted with a diagnosis of acute appendicitis and women contacted by a postal questionnaire.
2. The validity of case-control studies is questionable if the cases are not representative of the general population of women in their reproductive years who have PID.
3. Case-control studies do not measure the incidence or prevalence of PID among women using IUDs as contrasted to PID among women not using IUDs.

Investigators who conduct case-control studies have the advantage of being able to use existing data sources, such as hospital records. Certainly, case-control studies are easier, faster and more economical to perform than are prospective cohort studies. In the case of a rare event, the case-control approach may be the only feasible one. When available, however, the results of cohort studies are easier to interpret and have the distinct advantage of permitting computation of relative and attributable risk estimates of PID among IUD users versus nonusers.

Vessey and co-workers (96), in their prospective cohort study of women attending 17 clinics of the Family Planning Association in Great Britain, have presented evidence of an increased risk of PID among IUD users compared to nonusers (Table 4.1). The first episode rates of PID were significantly higher among IUD users than among nonusers for both in-patients (women admitted to a hospital for treatment) and for in-patients and out-patients (women treated at a hospital but not admitted). From this study, the excess rate of PID attributable to IUD use was estimated to be 1.45 additional cases of PID per 1,000 woman-years for in-patients. The corresponding rate for the in-patient/out-patient group was 1.65. These rates were standardized for age, parity, social class and smoking and may not be representative of the actual rates. If, however, the standardizing variables have little effect on the unadjusted hospitalization rate, then the rates reported by Vessey and co-workers (96) can be used to assess the excess rate of PID attributable to IUD use in the United Kingdom.

Kahn and Tyler (45) estimated the rate of IUD-related hospitalization to be 3 to 10 per 1,000 woman-years of IUD use, based on a mail survey of physicians likely to be involved with intrauterine contraception in the United States and Puerto Rico. Of the hospitalizations reported, 34.2% were for the treatment of a pelvic infection. Applying this percentage to the rate of 3 to 10 per 1,000 woman-years gives a rate of hospitalization for PID among IUD users of 1.0 to 3.4 per 1,000 woman-years. This rate is similar to the standardized rates of hospitalization given by Vessey and co-workers of 2.02 per 1,000 woman-years for IUD users. The rate for nonusers was 0.57 per 1,000 woman-years.

Regardless of the method of epidemiologic study, whether by the case-control or cohort approach, the clinical diagnosis of acute PID is subject to error. In recent years, the physician may be more likely to diagnose acute PID when evaluating a patient with clinical signs compatible with this diagnosis if it is known that the patient is an IUD user.

> A tentative diagnosis of PID in 23 Lippes Loop A and D users was confirmed in nine patients. Laboratory confirmation of PID could not be made in eight cases, and six women had other conditions (appendicitis, urinary tract infections, regional ileitis, postoperative wound infection with septicemia following a posterior colporraphy) (54).
> Jacobson and Westrom (41) reported that the clinical diagnosis of acute salpingitis was confirmed at laparoscopy or laparotomy in only 65.4% of the 814 cases. Twelve percent had other disorders; in 22.6% no specific diagnosis could be made.
> Feeney and El Badri (25) reported that among 48 women with a provisional diagnosis of acute PID, the diagnosis was confirmed at laparoscopy in 21 (43.8%) cases, was found incorrect in 7 (14.6%) cases and was indefinite in 20 (41.6%) cases.

A well-known study of IUD-related morbidity involving hospital in-patients was conducted by the National Center for Disease Control (CDC) in 1973 (45). The data from this survey were reanalyzed (44) to evaluate the apparent association between the Dalkon Shield and hospitalization rates for complicated pregnancies. This reanalysis revealed that 34.5% of the Dalkon Shield users, 30.4% of the Lippes Loop users and 32.6% of the Saf-T-Coil users were hospitalized with a diagnosis of pelvic infection. If women in the category "other and unknown diagnosis" (44) are excluded, the above percentages become 39.7, 37.3 and 39.8 respectively. Thus, among women who were hospitalized for an IUD-related complication, the proportions of Dalkon Shield, Lippes Loop and Saf-T-Coil users were not significantly different (p>.05). Nonetheless, it cannot be concluded that the risk of hospitalization for pelvic infection is the same for the three IUDs unless it is established that the rates of hospitalization for all reasons are similar for the three IUDs.

> Mosley and co-workers (65), in a reassessment of the data from the 1973 CDC study, concluded that after adjustments for duration of IUD use, the total hospitalization rate for the Dalkon Shield users was 4% to 18% higher than the rate for Lippes Loop and Saf-T-Coil users. They also concluded that there was no difference in the rates of hospitalization for women with complications not associated with pregnancy. Since hospitalizations for complicated pregnancy also could include hospitalizations for pelvic infection, the percentages of nonpregnant women who were hospitalized with a diagnosis of pelvic infection cannot be estimated from the data presented by Kahn and Tyler (44).

If the pregnancies which occur with the Dalkon Shield in situ are more likely to be complicated by sepsis, as has been suggested in some reports, then the available information (44,65) would indicate that among nonpregnant women, hospitalization rates for pelvic infection are not significantly different for users of the Dalkon Shield, the Lippes Loop and the Saf-T-Coil IUDs.

Most clinical and case reports do not provide sufficient data regarding the incidence of infection associated with IUD use to permit definite conclusions; nevertheless, they may provide information which implicates the IUD as a source of infection in individual patients.

> Mead and co-workers (61) reported on 63 patients with a diagnosis of acute PID who were admitted to the Gynecologic Service of a hospital which served

an isolated community of 24,795 women aged 15 to 44 years. There were 2,352 admissions over a two-year period. Twenty-six patients admitted with acute PID were using IUDs; 37 were not. The results of this study indicate that the incidence of PID requiring hospitalization was a rare event in this community, occurring in 0.25% of the women aged 15 to 44 years. Seven of the 26 women who were using IUDs underwent major operations as a direct result of IUD associated infections. No similar data were given for the nonuser group. The IUD insertion-to-infection interval was: 1 month, 14.3%; 2–12 months, 19.0%; 13–24 months, 23.8%; more than 24 months, 42.9%.

The following devices were present among the 26 hospitalized women with gynecological infections associated with an IUD: Dalkon Shield, 10 cases; Majzlin Spring, 4 cases; Copper T, 4 cases; Lippes Loop, 3 cases; IUD type unknown, 5 cases. In this study, the Dalkon Shield accounted for 38.5% (10/26) of the IUD-associated gynecological infections. This rate is similar to what one might expect considering that the Dalkon Shield accounted for 40% of all IUD sales in the study period (July 1972–June 1974). Four (15.4%) of the infections were associated with the Cu-T, an IUD which was not widely distributed during that time period.

The sales of the various types of IUDs in the community were not known at the time of the study, and Mead and co-workers (61) were unable to make any inferences regarding the relative rates of gynecological infections associated with the use of different IUDs. Furthermore, without knowledge of the number of women using IUDs, it is impossible to determine accurately the incidence of PID among IUD users or whether PID is more frequent among IUD users than among nonusers.

Although the various studies summarized in Table 4.1 provide evidence that IUD users in general

are at a higher risk of acquiring PID than are nonusers, we know of no comparative studies which
have specifically evaluated the relative incidence of
PID among women using different types of IUDs.
Therefore, current opinions as to whether or not
users of one type of IUD have a higher incidence of
PID are based either on incidental reports of PID
among women using different types of IUDs or PID
rates for specific IUDs reported in different studies.

Numerous studies reported in the literature
were reviewed to determine if there appear to be
significant differences in the rates of PID for different
types of IUDs. No evidence was found for a difference in the PID rates reported for different IUDs. This
is true not only for the IUDs inserted in the never
pregnant or not recently pregnant patient, but also
for IUDs inserted in patients immediately after an
abortion or at any time after a delivery. A sampling
of these studies has been summarized in Appendix
C. The studies are not necessarily representative of
all studies reviewed, but they have been summarized
to demonstrate the range of PID rates reported in different studies. Comparing the PID rates for different
types of IUDs from different studies is an unsatis-
factory method of evaluation for the following
reasons:

1. Often, no definition of PID was provided by the
   authors. Under these circumstances, the criteria
   for classifying an IUD-related problem as PID
   probably varied from investigator to investigator.
2. Most authors report PID rates as the percentage
   of patients with PID, which is not the best statistic for the comparison of PID rates associated
   with different IUDs. The percentage alone does
   not account for differing lengths of IUD use.
   Life table rates are preferable, but they were
   given in only a few studies.

Table 4.3 *PID rates (per 100 woman-years) for different types of IUDs.*

Months from Insertion	Lippes Loop, Birnberg Bow, Margulies Spiral, Steel Ring, Saf-T-Coil		Dalkon Shield		Progestasert	
	Woman-Years	PID Rate	Woman-Years	PID Rate	Woman-Years	PID Rate
≤ 1	1,882	5.8	185	5.4	511	8.0
2–12	16,144	2.6	1,468	2.5	3,700	3.5
13–24	10,588	2.2	728	2.5	—	—

3. Many of the studies reviewed did not even state PID rates, but rather presented removal rates for other medical reasons which included removals for PID, (e.g., Perlmutter [72], Herson and co-workers [38]). Other studies made no mention of the occurrence of PID or removals for PID.

Evidence to indicate that there are no significant differences among the PID rates for different IUDs may be obtained from the results of large multiclinic trials. The final report from the Cooperative Statistical Program (CSP) evaluated PID rates for several types of IUDs (95). There were no significant differences in the two-year PID rates per 100 women (net cumulative life-table rates) for the Lippes Loop (3.8), Margulies Sprial (3.6), Birnberg Bow (4.2), steel ring (4.1) and Saf-T-Coil (5.2). Of these IUDs, only the Lippes Loop and Saf-T-Coil are in widespread use today. Since the time of the report of Tietze and Lewit (95), other IUDs have been widely used, including the Dalkon Shield, Cu-7-200, Cu-T-200 and Progestasert. PID rates (per 100 woman-years) for the Dalkon Sheild (1), Progestasert (2) and for all IUDs reported in the CSP report (95) for various time periods from insertion are shown in Table 4.3. The PID rates for each time period from insertion are similar for the three multiclinic evaluations. The

PID rates shown in Table 4.3 include cases of suspected and confirmed PID. Data on PID rates from large-scale studies for users of copper-bearing IUDs were not available.

The PID rates for postpartum IUD insertions are generally higher than those for interval insertions. These higher rates, however, cannot necessarily be attributed to the IUD, since endometritis is more common after termination of pregnancy, even without IUD insertion.

Studies which have evaluated the risks associated with the immediate postabortal insertion of an IUD are summarized and discussed in Chapter 2. None of the studies reviewed reported an increased risk of PID among women who had postabortal IUD insertions. In fact, some of the studies suggested that there may be a decreased risk of septic complications for women who have a postabortal IUD insertion compared to those women who do not have a postabortal IUD insertion.

Tubo-Ovarian Abscess

Tubo-ovarian abscess is one of the most serious forms of PID and carries the risk of rupture and subsequent generalized peritonitis, sepsis and death. Several authors have reported an association between IUD use and tubo-ovarian or pelvic abscess, and some authors have inferred that unilateral tubo-ovarian abscesses may occur more frequently among IUD users than among nonusers.

Wilson and Dilts (103) reported on two unilateral tubo-ovarian abscesses; one occurred two months after insertion of a Dalkon Shield and the other 15 months after insertion of a Lippes Loop.

Duckman and co-workers (20) reported two cases of tubo-ovarian abscess following insertion of

a Majzlin Spring. The first, a bilateral abscess, occurred 1.5 years after insertion; the second, a unilateral abscess, occurred 2.5 years after insertion.

Golditch and Huston (30) noted tubo-ovarian
and pelvic abscesses which occurred four weeks to
five years after IUD insertion. The devices used were
Majzlin Springs (4 women), Lippes Loops (3 women)
and Dalkon Shields (3 women). The type of IUD was
unknown in seven cases.

Beecham and co-workers (6) reported three cases
of bilateral tubo-ovarian abscesses occurring 11 to 30
months after insertion of Majzlin Springs.

Dawood and Birnbaum (18) reported on four unilateral tubo-ovarian abscesses (Dalkon Shield, 3;
Lippes Loop, 1). The Dalkon Shield patients were
treated one year after insertion; the Lippes Loop patient was treated nine months after insertion.

Sixteen cases of unilateral tubo-ovarian abscesses, pyosalpinx or ovarian abscesses in association
with IUD use were reported by Taylor and co-
workers (92). Nine patients were using a shield type
IUD, 4 a Lippes Loop, 1 a Saf-T-Coil, 1 a spring device and 1 a copper device. The time from IUD insertion ranged from less than one month to over four
years.

Kostelnik and Fremount (49) reported on a case
of a unilateral tubo-ovarian abscess 11 years after
the insertion of a Lippes Loop.

Golde and co-workers (29) reported on 85 tubo-
ovarian abscesses of which 32 (38%) were associated
with IUD use. Of the 37 unilateral tubo-ovarian abscesses, 20 (54.1%) were associated with IUD use,
compared to 25.0% of the 48 bilateral tubo-ovarian
abscesses. Twenty users of the Dalkon Shield accounted for 62.5% of the abscesses. The remaining
women had Lippes Loops (9 women), Saf-T-Coil
(1 woman) or Cu-T devices (2 women). Among the
IUD users with a unilateral or bilateral tubo-ovarian
abscess, the Dalkon Shield was associated with 65%

of the unilateral and 58% of the bilateral abscesses.
The duration of IUD use ranged from 1 to 5 years
(mean, 2.3 years) for the Dalkon Shield users, 3 days
to 6 years (mean, 2.5 years) for the Lippes Loop users,
3 months for the Saf-T-Coil user and 3 months and 1
year for the two Cu-T-200 users.

Scott (81) reviewed 46 cases of tubo-ovarian
abscesses of which 28.3% were IUD-associated, and
20 cases of pelvic abscesses of which 30% were IUD-
related. Among the IUD users, tubo-ovarian abscesses were bilateral in 5 cases and unilateral in
8 cases.

Kanter (47), Wright (105) and Badra and co-
workers (5) summarized 5 cases of tubo-ovarian
abscesses following laparoscopic tubal cauterization
and IUD removal.

Golditch and Huston (30) provide evidence
which suggests that IUD users are not at any greater
risk of tubo-ovarian and/or pelvic abscesses than are
nonusers. Bacteriologic studies of endometrial
swabs were made for 235 patients seen for gynecological examination. Of these patients, 55.7% were
IUD users. Over a 30-month period, 31 women were
admitted with a diagnosis of tubo-ovarian abscess
(22 women) or pelvic abscess (9 women). Of these 31
women, 17 (54.8%) were IUD users. Thirteen
(59.1%) of the tubo-ovarian abscesses occurred in
IUD users. If it is assumed that the 235 patients who
had endometrial cultures were not preselected on
the basis of contraceptive methods used, then the
similarity of the percentage of patients seen for gynecological examination who were IUD users (55.7%)
and the percentage of patients with tubo-ovarian abscess (54.5%) or pelvic abscesses who were IUD
users (57.8%) suggests that the incidence of tubo-
ovarian and/or pelvic abscesses is no different for
IUD users and nonusers. No other published studies
provided the necessary data to determine whether

or not IUD users are at a higher risk of tubo-ovarian and/or pelvic abscesses than are nonusers.

Recently, actinomycosis infections of the genital tract have been reported in association with tubo-ovarian abscess among IUD users.

> Forty-three cases of actinomycosis infections associated with IUD use have been reported (Cu-7, 2 cases; Lippes Loop, 9 cases; Majzlin Spring, 19 cases; Birnberg Bow, 1 case; Dalkon Shield, 8 cases; Saf-T-Coil, 2 cases; endocervical contraceptive device, 1 case; vaginal pessary, 1 case) (8,19,36,56,59,64,75,78, 79,89,104). Among these 43 cases, 14 (32.6%) had tubo-ovarian abscesses (7 unilateral, 7 bilateral).

Although only about 300 cases of pelvic actinomycosis had been reported in the literature as of 1972, this organism may be more prevalent than previously suspected. Gupta and co-workers (33) have identified *Actinomyces isreaeli* and *Actinomyces naeslundi* in nearly 200 Papanicolaou-stained (fast) cervico-vaginal smears. More recently, Spence and co-workers (86) have identified these organisms in the Papanicolaou-stained smears of 35 IUD users, 20% of whom were asymptomatic.

Some authors (18,92) have hypothesized that trauma to the endometrium caused by embedding of the IUD or by other means may create a path of infection from the vagina to the endometrium and myometrium and may support a further spread to the uterine tubes through the parametrium. If this hypothesis is true, then a higher incidence of tubo-ovarian abscesses would be expected among women using devices that embed into the uterus or cause trauma to the endometrium.

A number of investigators have suggested that the lateral projections of the Dalkon Shield may cause trauma to the endometrium. The Majzlin Spring and the M IUD (both made from stainless

steel) are frequently embedded into the endometrium. Hysterographic studies have shown that retention of the Cu-T is facilitated by the embedding of
the tip(s) of the transverse arm into the endometrium
(46,48). Retention of the Cu-7 probably is facilitated
by a similar mechanism.

Case Reports

Although numerous fatalities and serious infectious
complications have been reported in the literature
(12,14,17,28,31,37,39,43,58,76,80,93,97,99), these
case reports neither provide estimates of the rate of
infectious complications associated with IUD use,
nor establish a causal relationship between IUD use
and the type of complication. The case reports,
however, do serve to indicate the extent and variation of the problems that may be encountered
among IUD users.

Summary

This chapter has reviewed reports regarding the
association between the use of intrauterine devices
and the occurrence of PID. Bacteriologic studies
suggest that a transient bacteriologic contamination
of the endometrial cavity occurs after IUD insertion.
Histopathologic studies show variable rates of a
chronic inflammatory response, with consistently
higher rates of chronic endometritis among women
who have their IUDs removed because of IUD-
related symptoms (abnormal bleeding, pain, discharge) than among asymptomatic women who
have their IUDs removed.

Epidemiologic studies suggest that there is an
increased risk of acute PID among IUD users compared to nonusers. From the available data, it ap-

pears that the rate of hospitalization for PID among IUD users ranges from 1.0 to 3.4 per 1,000 woman-years of IUD use.

Some of the variations seen in the reported rates of PID may be attributed to varying diagnostic criteria used by the investigators, different incidence rates of PID in the geographic locale where the investigation took place, and differences in the method(s) of reporting PID rates. In the great majority of instances, the only proportions reported were for women using IUDs who acquired PID. In most studies, the life-table method of reporting, which takes into account varying durations of patient observation, was absent. Life-table rates could not be calculated from the data obtained from the literature. There is conflicting evidence as to whether or not nulliparous IUD users are at a higher risk of PID compared to parous IUD users. If there is an increased risk for the nulliparous IUD user, the magnitude of the risk appears to be small.

Our review of IUD studies indicates similar rates of PID for all types of commercially available IUDs. While there does appear to be an increased risk of PID among IUD users compared to nonusers, the magnitude of increased risk remains uncertain.

References

1. A. H. Robins Company. Unpublished data. Richmond, Virginia.

2. Alza Corporation, *The Progestasert*. Intrauterine progesterone contraceptive system release rated 65 μg/day progesterone for one year. Alza Product Information, Palo Alto, California, 1977.

3. Anonymous. Dangers of Gomco intra-uterine silver rings. *JAMA* 108:413, 1937.

4. Anonymous. Ob-Gyn panel recommends PID warning label for IUDs: keeps CO_2 lasers in premarket. *Medical Devices Report* Vol. V, no. L, June 16, 1977.

5. Badra, P. L.; Young, J. R.; Laros, R. K.; and Peterson, E. P. Suppurative salpingitis after laparoscopic tubal cauterization. *Obstet. Gynecol.* 42:511, 1973.

6. Beecham, J. B.; Maeck, J. V. S.; and Mead, P. B. Severe pelvic sepsis and the Majzlin Spring. *Obstet. Gynecol.* 43:159, 1974.

7. Berger, G. S.; Keith, L.; and Moss, W. Prevalence of gonorrhea among women using various methods of contraception. *Br. J. Vener. Dis.* 51:307, 1975.

8. Brenner, R. W., and Gehring, S. W. Pelvic actinomycosis in the presence of an endocervical contraceptive device. Report of a case. *Obstet. Gynecol.* 29:71, 1967.

9. Buchman, M. I. A study of the intrauterine contraceptive device with and without an extracervical appendage or tail. *Fertil. Steril.* 21:348, 1970.

10. Burnhill, M. S. Syndrome of progressive endometritis associated with intrauterine contraceptive devices. *Adv. Plann. Parent.* 8:144, 1973.

11. Chow, A. W.; Malkasian, L.; Marshall, J. R.; and Guze, L. B. The bacteriology of acute pelvic inflammatory disease. Value of cul-de-sac cultures and relative importance of gonococci and other aerobic or anaerobic bacteria. *Am. J. Obstet. Gynec.* 122:876, 1975.

12. Cobbs, C. G. IUD and endocarditis. *Ann. Int. Med.* 78:451, 1973.

13. Cohen, L., and Thomas, G. Copper versus the gonococcus *in vivo. Br. J. Vener. Dis.* 50:364, 1974.

14. Colin, M. J., and Weissman, G. Disseminated gonococcal infection and tenosynovitis from an asymp-
tomatically infected intrauterine contraceptive device. *N. Engl. J. Med.* 294:598, 1976.

15. Combined Bangkok Hospital Group and Wright,
N. H. Unsuspected pelvic infection discovered at
tubal ligation: relationship to use of intrauterine
contraception. In *Analysis of intrauterine devices*,
eds. F. Hefnawi and S. J. Segal. New York: American
Elsevier Publishing Co., Inc., 1975.

16. Cornfield, J. A method of estimating comparative
rates from clinical data. Applications to cancer of
the lung, breast, and cervix. *J. Natl. Can. Inst.* 11:
1269, 1951.

17. Culliford, A. T.; Harris, M. N.; Porges, R. F.; Berczel-
ler, P. H.; Amorosi, E. L.; and Grier, W. R. N. Strep-
tococcal peritonitis in a patient with Hodgkin's Disease and an intrauterine contraceptive device. *Am. J.
Obstet. Gynecol.* 117:288, 1973.

18. Dawood, M. Y., and Birnbaum, S. J. Unilateral tubo-
ovarian abscess and intrauterine contraceptive device. *Obstet. Gynecol.* 46:429, 1975.

19. Dische, F. E.; Burt, J. M.; Davidson, J. H.; and Pun-
tambekar, S. Tubo-ovarian actinomycosis associated
with intrauterine contraceptive devices. *J. Obst.
Gynaec. Brit. Comnwlth.* 81:724, 1974.

20. Duckman, S.; Suarez, J.; and Tantakesem, P. Tubo-
ovarian abscess and the intrauterine device (Majzlin
Spring). *Am. J. Obstet. Gynecol.* 115:1157, 1973.

21. Elstein, M. Pelvic inflammation and the intrauterine
contraceptive device. *Proc. Roy. Soc. Med.* 60:397,
1967.

22. Eschenbach, D. A.; Harnisch, J. P.; and Holmes, K. K.
Pathogenesis of acute pelvic inflammatory disease:

role of contraception and other risk factors. *Am. J. Obstet. Gynecol.* 128:838, 1977.

23. Eschenbach, D. A., and Holmes, K. K. Acute pelvic inflammatory disease: current concepts of pathogenesis, etiology, and management. *Clin. Obstet. Gynecol.* 18:35, 1975.

24. Faulkner, W. L., and Ory, H. W. Intrauterine devices and acute pelvic inflammatory disease. *JAMA* 235: 1851, 1976.

25. Feeney, J. G., and El Badri, A. Screening for gonococcal salpingitis. *Lancet* 2:1309, 1976.

26. Fiscina, B.; Oster, G. K.; Oster, G.; and Swanson, J. Gonococcicidal action of copper *in vitro*. *Am. J. Obstet. Gynecol.* 116:86, 1973.

27. Fleiss, J. *Statistical methods for rates and proportions.* New York: John Wiley and Sons, 1973.

28. Gallant, T. E.; Malinak, L. R.; Gump, D. W.; and Mead, P. B. Hemophilus parainfluenzae peritonitis associated with an intrauterine contraceptive device. *Am. J. Obstet. Gynecol.* 129:702, 1977.

29. Golde, S. H.; Israel, R.; and Ledger; W. J. Unilateral tubo-ovarian abscess: a distinct entity. *Am. J. Obstet. Gynecol.* 127:807, 1977.

30. Golditch, I. M., and Huston, J. E. Serious pelvic infections associated with intrauterine contraceptive device. *Int. J. Fertil.* 18:156, 1973.

31. Goldman, J. A. Infected ovarian cysts and the IUD. *Contraception* 8:521, 1973.

32. Gray, R. Pelvic inflammatory disease and intrauterine contraceptive devices. *Lancet* 2:521, 1976.

33. Gupta, P. K.; Hollander, D. H.; and Frost, J. K. Acti-

nomycetes in cervico-vaginal smears: an association with IUD usage. *Acta Cytol.* 20:295, 1976.

34. Hagenfeldt, K. Intrauterine contraception with the Copper-T device. 1. Effect on trace elements in the endometrium, cervical mucus and plasma. *Contraception* 6:37, 1972.

35. Hager, W. D., and Wiesner, P. J. Selected epidemiologic aspects of acute salpingitis: a review. *J. Reprod. Med.* 19:47, 1977.

36. Henderson, S. R. Pelvic actinomycosis associated with an intrauterine device. *Obstet. Gynecol.* 41: 726, 1973.

37. Herbert, T. J., and Mortimer, P. P. Recurrent pneumococcal peritonitis associated with an intra-uterine contraceptive device. *Br. J. Surg.* 61:901, 1974.

38. Herson, J.; Crocker, C. L.; and Butts, E. Loop vs. shield: a competing risks analysis of IUD termination. *Contraception* 14:67, 1976.

39. Hurley, R. Haemophilus endometritis in woman fitted with Lippes Loop. *Br. Med. J.* 1:566, 1970.

40. Israel, R., and Davis, H. J. Effect of intrauterine contraceptive devices on the endometrium. *JAMA* 195: 144, 1966.

41. Jacobson, L., and Westrom, L. Objectivized diagnosis of acute pelvic inflammatory disease. Diagnostic and prognostic value of routine laparoscopy. *Am. J. Obstet. Gynecol.* 105:1088, 1969.

42. Johannisson, G.; Karamustafa, A.; and Brorson, J-E. Influence of copper salts on gonococci. *Br. J. Vener. Dis.* 52:176, 1976.

43. Kahn, H. S., and Tyler, C. W. Mortality associated with the use of IUDs. *JAMA* 234:57, 1975.

44. Kahn, H. S., and Tyler, C. W. An association between the Dalkon Shield and complicated pregnancies among women hospitalized for intrauterine contraceptive device-related disorders. *Am. J. Obstet. Gynecol.* 125:83, 1976.

45. Kahn, H. S., and Tyler, C. W. IUD-related hospitalizations in United States and Puerto Rico, 1973. *JAMA* 234:53, 1975.

46. Kamal, I.; Ghoneim, M.; Talaat, M.; and Mallawani, A. The anchoring mechanism of retention of the Copper T device. *Fertil. Steril.* 24:165, 1973.

47. Kanter, E. Tubo-ovarian abscess associated with laparoscopic tubal cauterization and the intrauterine contraceptive device. *Am. J. Obstet. Gynecol.* 121:291, 1975.

48. Khatamee, M. A., and Lehfeldt, H. Hysterographic studies in women wearing Copper-T devices. *Adv. Plann. Parent.* X:90, 1975.

49. Kostelnik, F. V., and Fremount, H. N. Mycotic tubo-ovarian abscess associated with the intrauterine device. *Am. J. Obstet. Gynecol.* 125:272, 1976.

50. Kulka, E. W.; Lehfeldt, H.; and Getmanov-Von der Mosel, V. Adverse experience with stainless steel spring intrauterine device. *N. Y. State J. Med.* p. 694, March 15, 1972.

51. Ledger, W. J. Relationship of pelvic infection to various types of contraception. *Clin. Obstet. Gynecol.* 17:79, 1974.

52. Lee, C. H.; Chow, L. P.; Cheng, T. Y.; and Wei, P. Y. Histologic study of the endometrium of intrauterine contraceptive device users. *Am. J. Obstet. Gynecol.* 98:808, 1967.

53. Lip, J., and Burgoyne, X. Cervical and peritoneal bac-

terial flora associated with salpingitis. *Obstet. Gynecol.* 28:561, 1966.

54. Lippes, J. Contraception with intrauterine plastic loops. *Am. J. Obstet. Gynecol.* 93:1024, 1965.

55. Lippes, J. Infection and the IUD: a preliminary report. *Contraception* 12:103, 1975.

56. Lomax, C. W.; Harbert, G. M.; and Thornton, W. N. Actinomycosis of the female genital tract. *Obstet. Gynecol.* 48:341, 1976.

57. Mardh, P-A., and Westrom, L. Tubal and cervical cultures in acute salpingitis with special reference to mycoplasma hominis and T-strain mycoplasmas. *Br. J. Vener. Dis.* 46:179, 1970.

58. Marshall, B. R.; Hepler, J. K.; and Jinguji, M. S. Fatal streptococcus pyogenes septicemia associated with an intrauterine device. *Obstet. Gynecol.* 41:83, 1973.

59. McCormick, J. F., and Scorgie, R. D. F. Unilateral tubo-ovarian actinomycosis in the presence of an intrauterine device. *Am. J. Clin. Pathol.* 68:622, 1977.

60. McCormack, W. M.; Johnson, K.; Stumacher, R. J.; Donner, A.; and Rychwalski, R. Clinical spectrum of gonococcal infection in women. *Lancet* 1:1182, 1977.

61. Mead, P. B.; Beecham, J. B.; and Maeck, J. V. S. Incidence of infections associated with the intrauterine contraceptive device in an isolated community. *Am. J. Obstet. Gynecol.* 125:79, 1976.

62. Miettinen, O. Simple interval-estimation of risk ratio. *Am. J. Epidem.* 100:515, 1974.

63. Mishell, D. R.; Bell, J. H.; Good, R. G.; and Moyer, D. L. The intrauterine device: a bacteriologic study

of the intrauterine cavity. *Am. J. Obstet. Gynecol.* 96:119, 1966.

64. Mittal, S.; Mukerjee, A.; and Monga, J. N. Bilateral actinomycosis of the ovaries. *J. Obstet. Gynaecol.* (India) XXIII:517, 1973.

65. Mosley, W. H.; Chow, L. P.; and Liu, P. T. IUD related hospitalizations. A further analysis of device specific associations in the 1973 CDC study. Unpublished report from the Department of Population Dynamics. Johns Hopkins University, Baltimore, Maryland.

66. Moyer, D. L., and Mishell, D. R. Reactions of human endometrium to the intrauterine foreign body. II. Long-term effects on the endometrial histology and cytology. *Am. J. Obstet. Gynecol.* 111:66, 1971.

67. Noonan, A. S., and Adams, J. B. Gonorrhea screening in an urban hospital family planning program. *Am. J. Pub. Health* 64:700, 1974.

68. Ober, W. B.; Sobrero, A. J.; and De Chabon, A. B. Endometrial findings after insertion of stainless steel spring IUD. *Obstet. Gynecol.* 36:62, 1970.

69. Ober, W. B.; Sobrero, A. J.; De Chabon, A. B.; and Goodman, J. Polyethylene intrauterine contraceptive device. Endometrial changes following long-term use. *JAMA* 212:765, 1970.

70. Ober, W. B.; Sobrero, A. J.; Kurman, R.; and Gold, S. Endometrial morphology and polyethylene intrauterine devices. A study of 200 endometrial biopsies. *Obstet. Gynecol.* 32:782, 1968.

71. Osser, S.; Gallberg, B.; Liedholm, P.; and Sjoberg, N-O. Is development of pelvic inflammatory disease in women using intra-uterine devices equal regardless of parity? A one year follow-up study. *Contraception* 17:563, 1978.

72. Perlmutter, J. F. Experience with the Dalkon Shield as a contraceptive device. *Obstet. Gynecol.* 43:443, 1974.

73. Phaosavasdi, S.; Vivanichakul, B.; Rienprayura, D.; Chutivongse, S.; Virutamasen, P.; and Snidvongs, W. Pelvic inflammatory disease in contraceptive acceptors disclosed at transvaginal tubal sterilization. In *Analysis of intrauterine devices*, eds. F. Hefnawi and S. J. Segal. New York: American Elsevier Publishing Co., Inc., 1975.

74. Philips, F.; Arumugam, K.; and Prema, K. Clinical and histopathological picture in long term loop-study of 170 cases at Government Erskine Hospital, Madurai, Tamilnadu, India. In *Proceedings of the 6th Asian Congress of Obstetrics and Gynaecology*, ed. T. A. Sinnathuray. Kuala Lumpur, Malaysia, 1974.

75. Purdie, D. W.; Carty, M. J.; and McLeod, T. I. F. Tubo-ovarian actinomycosis and the IUCD. *Br. Med. J.* 2:1392, 1977.

76. Rowland, T. C. Severe peritonitis complicating an intrauterine contraceptive device. *Am. J. Obstet. Gynecol.* 110:786, 1971.

77. Salmi, T.; Jarvinen, H.; Rauramo, L.; and Timonen, H. Cervical bacterial flora in women fitted with a copper-releasing intra-uterine contraceptive device (IUD). *Acta Obstet. Gynecol.*. (Scand) 55:317, 1976.

78. Schiffer, M. A.; Elguezabal, A.; Sultana, M.; and Allen, A. C. Actinomycosis infections associated with intrauterine contraceptive devices. *Obstet. Gynecol.* 45:67, 1975.

79. Schiffer, M. A.; Elguezabal, A.; and Allen, A. C. Actinomycosis infections associated with intrauterine contraceptive devices and a vaginal pessary. *Adv. Plann. Parent.* 12:183, 1978.

80. Scott, R. B. A survey of deaths and critical illnesses in association with the use of intrauterine devices. *Int. J. Fertil.* 13:297, 1968.

81. Scott, W. C. Pelvic abscess in association with intrauterine contraceptive device. *Am. J. Obstet. Gynecol.* 131:149, 1978.

82. Sen, R.; Ray, K.; Bose, C.; Kripalani, G.; and Purkayastha, N. An assessment of the safety of inserting Lippes' "loop" as intrauterine contraceptive device in respect to microbial infection. *Indian J. Med. Res.* 56:668, 1968.

83. Smith, M. R., and Soderstrom, R. Salpingitis: a frequent response to intrauterine contraception. *J. Reprod. Med.* 16:159, 1976.

84. Sparks, R. A.; Purrier, B. G. A.; Watt, P. J.; and Elstein, M. The bacteriology of the cervical canal in relation to the use of an intrauterine contraceptive device. Paper presented at The Uterine Cervix in Reproduction Workshop Conference, 24–26, June 1977, Rottach-Egern, West Germany.

85. Spellacy, W. N.; Hiser, B. J.; and Birk, S. A. The effect of copper intrauterine devices on endocervical gonococcal cultures. *Fertil. Steril.* 25:772, 1974.

86. Spence, M. R.; Gupta, P. K.; Frost, J. K.; and King, T. M. Cytologic detection and clinical significance of *Actinomycoses israelii* in women using intrauterine contraceptive devices. *Am. J. Obstet. Gynecol.* 131: 295, 1978.

87. Spence, M. R.; Stutz, D. R.; and Paniom, W. Effect of a copper-containing intrauterine contraceptive device on *Neisseria gonorrhoeae in vitro. Am. J. Obstet. Gynecol.* 122:783, 1975.

88. Statham, R., and Morton, R. S. Gonorrhea and the intrauterine contraceptive device. *Br. Med. J.* 4:623, 1968.

89. Surur, F. Actinomycosis of female genital tract. *N. Y. State J. Med.* 408, 1974.

90. Targum, S. D., and Wright, N. H. Association of the intrauterine device and pelvic inflammatory disease: a retrospective pilot study. *Am. J. Epidem.* 100:262, 1974.

91. Tatum, H. J.; Schmidt, F. H.; Phillips, D.; McCarty, M.; and O'Leary, W. M. The Dalkon Shield controversy: structural and bacteriological studies of IUD tails. *JAMA* 231:711, 1975.

92. Taylor, E. S.; McMillan, J. H.; Greer, B. E.; Droegemueller, W.; and Thompson, H. E. The intrauterine device and tubo-ovarian abscess. *Am. J. Obstet. Gynecol.* 123:338, 1975.

93. Taylor, K. C. G. A death directly attributable to the insertion of an IUD. *J. Fam. Plann. Doctors* 2:61, 1977.

94. Thaler, I.; Paldi, E.; and Steiner, D. Intrauterine device and pelvic inflammatory disease. *Int. J. Fertil.* 23:69, 1978.

95. Tietze, C., and Lewit, S. Evaluation of intrauterine devices: ninth progress report of the Cooperative Statistical Program. *Stud. Fam. Plann.* 59:July, 1970.

96. Vessey, M.; Doll, R.; Peto, R.; Johnson, B.; and Wiggins, P. A long-term follow-up study of women using different methods of contraception—an interim report. *J. Biosoc. Sci.* 8:383, 1976.

97. Weiland, A. J.; Tarzy, B. J.; and Young, P. E. Ligneous cellulitis associated with an IUD. *Obstet. Gynecol.* 51:48S, 1978 (Supplement).

98. Westrom, L.; Bengstsson, L. P.; and Mardh, P. A. The risk of pelvic inflammatory disease in women using

intrauterine contraceptive devices as compared to non-users. *Lancet* 2:221, 1976.

99. Wiknjostro, H.; Doodoh, A.; Rachman, I.; Agussja-ries, Harap H.; Mitra, M.; and Thomas, M. Post-partum use of the Lippes Loop and Dalkon Shield. In *Proceedings of the Asian Federation of Obstetrics and Gynaecology*, 1st Inter-Congress, Singapore, 1976. Singapore: Asian Federation of Obstetrics and Gynaecology, 1976.

100. Willson, J. R.; Bollinger, C. C.; and Ledger, W. J. The effect of an intrauterine contraceptive device on the bacterial flora of the endometrial cavity. *Am. J. Obstet. Gynecol.* 90:726, 1964.

101. Willson, J. R.; Ledger, W. J.; Andros, G. J.; and Bol-linger, C. C. Genital tract infection with an intra-uterine contraceptive device: a histopathologic study. In *Proceedings of the 2nd International Con-ference on Contraception*, New York, 1964. Amster-dam: Excerpta Medica Series, no. 86, 1964.

102. Willson, J. R.; Ledger, W. J.; Bollinger, C. C.; and Andros, G. J. The Margulies intrauterine contracep-tive device. Experience with 623 women. *Am. J. Obstet. Gynecol.* 112:237, 1972.

103. Wilson, E. A., and Dilts, P. V. Unusual complica-tion of an intrauterine contraceptive device. *Am. J. Obstet. Gynecol.* 122:237, 1972.

104. Witwer, M. W.; Farmer, M. F.; Wand, J. S.; and Solo-mon, L. S. Extensive actinomycosis associated with tion of an intrauterine contraceptive device. *Am. J. Obstet. Gynecol.* 121:237, 1972.

105. Wright, F. C. Tubo-ovarian abscess associated with laparoscopic tubal cauterization and the intrauterine contraceptive device. *Am. J. Obstet. Gynecol.* 119: 1133, 1974.

106. Wright, N. H., and Laemmle, P. Acute pelvic inflam-

matory disease in an indigent population. An estimate of the incidence and relationship to methods of contraception. *Am. J. Obstet.Gynecol.* 101:979, 1968.

Chapter 5

Bleeding

Introduction

A review of the pertinent literature shows that bleeding and/or pain represent the most frequently given reasons for IUD removal. Unfortunately, these two conditions are usually reported as a single entity, and this does not permit calculation of the true removal rate for bleeding alone. Another factor which limits an assessment of the extent of IUD-associated bleeding is that removal of the IUD is often performed on the basis of subjective judgments by women and/or their physicians regarding the amount of blood lost.

Quantitative Analysis of Blood Loss

Those studies which have quantitatively evaluated the extent of IUD-associated bleeding have separated bleeding into three distinct and quantifiable categories: 1) amount of menstrual blood loss (flow), 2) duration of menstrual blood loss and 3) occurrence of intermenstrual bleeding.

Amount of Menstrual Blood Loss

The studies which have quantitatively evaluated menstrual blood loss (MBL) after IUD insertion show

significant increases in the amount of blood loss for
all IUDs except for those which release progesterone.
These reports are summarized in Table 5.1. Variations in MBL as reported in different studies are
probably related to differences in: 1) groups of wom-
en studied, 2) instructions provided and methods
used to collect the menstrual flow, 3) methods used
to measure the blood collected and 4) types of IUD.

The larger nonmedicated IUDs are associated
with a higher mean MBL than the smaller copper-
bearing IUDs. Apparently, the smaller increase in
MBL for copper-bearing IUDs is not a result of any
local effect of the copper on the endometrium, but is
due to the reduced size of these IUDs. Hefnawi and
co-workers (9) reported that the mean MBLs were
not significantly different for women who used a
Lippes Loop D with or without copper.

There is no agreement as to whether the mean
MBL decreases with increased duration of IUD use
for nonmedicated and copper-bearing IUDs. The apparent decrease in the mean MBL observed in some
studies may result from the methods of data analysis.
Women may discontinue IUD use for a number of
reasons, including IUD removal for bleeding problems. Analyses of MBL among the continuing
users would give a better indication of whether there
were significant changes over time. Unfortunately,
this type of analytical approach was not followed in
any of the studies listed in Table 5.1.

In contrast to what may be expected, women
with documented preinsertion histories of menorrhagia (defined as a menstrual blood loss of over 80
ml per cycle) have a proportionally smaller increase
in MBL than do women with a "normal" preinsertion MBL. Among women with normal MBLs before
IUD insertion, the mean post-IUD insertion MBL
increases by 80% or more (Table 5.1) for women
who have a nonmedicated or copper-bearing IUD
inserted.

Malmquist and co-workers (19) inserted Cu-T IUDs in 16 women with "profuse menstruations." Their mean preinsertion MBL was 97 ml compared to mean postinsertion losses of 113, 103 and 103 ml at 1, 2 and 3 months, respectively. In four menorrhagic women with a MBL of 106 to 160 ml in eight pre-insertion cycles, there was a decrease in blood loss in 12 of 16 menstrual cycles following the insertion of a Cu-7.

The effect of parity on MBL in association with IUD use is uncertain.

Rybo (28) demonstrated that MBL was not related to the woman's parity.

Liedholm and co-workers (17) showed no dif-ferences in the mean MBL for nulliparas and multi-paras, either before or after insertion of Cu-T IUDs.

Guillebaud and co-workers (5) found that the MBL was lower for nulliparas than for multiparas both before and after the insertion of Dalkon Shields or Cu-7s.

Progesterone-releasing devices, in contrast to other IUDs, appear to reduce the MBL volume from its preinsertion level. This apparently results from suppression of endometrial growth by the proges-terone.

Rybo (29) reported that the Progestasert was associ-ated with a 25% reduction in the MBL by three months after insertion as compared with preinsertion cycles.

The World Health Organization (34) reported a 45% decrease in preinsertion MBL among Progesta-sert users by 12 months after insertion.

Martinez-Manautou and co-workers (20) studied 367 women who complained of profuse menstrual bleeding prior to Progestasert insertions. Only 18%

Table 5.1 Summary of studies which have quantitatively evaluated menstrual blood loss (MBL) associated with IUD use.

| Reference Number | IUD | Number of Subjects | Preinsertion | Mean MBL (ml) Postinsertion (months) | | | | | Menorrhagia (Percentage) | Comments |
				1	3	6	12	All		
33	Saf-T-Coil 33S	31	35.8	78.2	57.3	•	•	65.4	42.2	Menorrhagia = MBL > 60 ml. % with menorrhagia is the percentage of cycles, not subjects.
6	Birnberg Bow Antigon }	20	35.5	66.6	82.2	•	•	73.1	•	•
8	Cu-T-200 }	91	•	62.2	50.8	42.0	37.0	47.8	•	Mean MBL from 145 untreated controls: 37 ml.
	Cu-7-200									
	Lippes Loop C	50	•	•	•	•	•	78.0	•	
10	Lippes Loop D	72	•	•	•	75.0	56.5	66.6	47.0	Menorrhagia = MBL > 60 ml. Mean MBL among 19 noncontraceptive menses: 34.6 ml; incidence of menorrhagia: 5.3%.
	Dalkon Shield	73	•	•	•	60.4	74.7	67.5	44.0	
	Cu-T-200	83	•	•	•	54.5	55.2	53.1	33.0	
16	Saf-T-Coil	10	•	•	•	•	•	45.0	•	Mean MBL in a control group of women was 21 ml.
	Dalkon Shield	9	•	•	•	•	•	62.0	•	
	Cu-7-200	10	•	•	•	•	•	30.0	•	

Ref.	Device	No.						Incidence	Comments
21	Cu-T-200	9	38.1	66.0	85.0	•	73.0	•	
	T releasing 25 µg/day d-norgestrel	10	52.3	32.2	18.5	•	21.0	•	
19	Cu-T-200	50	37.2	56.1	44.8	•	53.6	•	
	Cu-7-200	16	35.7	44.4	38.8	•	39.7	•	
12	Lippes Loop D	28	42.7	121.1	93.5	89.5	•	•	
14	Cu-7-200	43	36.3	54.3	58.4	58.8	57.1	18.8	Menorrhagia = MBL > 80 ml. Incidence of menorrhagia based on cycles, not subjects.
17	Cu-T-200 nulliparas	18	29.3	56.0	62.4	62.9	41.3	46.0 ⎫	Menorrhagia = MBL > 80 ml.
	Cu-T-200 multiparas	24	31.8	65.2	44.2	49.0	57.8	⎭	
5	Lippes Loop D	76	41.0	•	•	•	90.0	51.0	Multiparas. Menorrhagia = MBL > 80 ml. Only 14% had menorrhagia preinsertion. Nulliparas
	Dalkon Shield (standard)	70	46.0	•	•	•	81.0	41.0	
	Cu-7-200	91	45.0	•	•	•	63.0	25.0	
	Dalkon Shield (small)	18	18.0	•	•	•	46.0	•	
	Cu-7-200	24	16.0	•	•	•	36.0	•	

Table 5.1 (cont'd)

Reference Number	IUD	Number of Subjects	Preinsertion	Mean MBL (ml) Postinsertion (months)					Menorrhagia (Percentage)	Comments
				1	3	6	12	All		
7	Lippes Loop C	14	•	•	•	•	•	⎫	•	•
	Saf-T-Coil	2	•	•	•	•	•	⎬ 65.0	•	•
	Dalkon Shield	1	•	•	•	•	•	⎪	•	•
	Cu-7	1	•	•	•	•	•	⎭	•	•
9	Lippes Loop D	44	24.1	63.7	53.8	37.7	28.3	•	•	•
	Lippes Loop D with copper	37	29.6	68.3	60.2	45.8	33.8	•	•	•
4	Cu-T-220C	8	24.4	47.9	80.0	76.1	•	•	•	•
	Cu-T-380B	12	57.0	108.6	100.3	90.1	•	•	•	•
	Cu-T-200	14	33.6	64.7	65.5	63.7	•	•	•	•
	Lippes Loop D	11	69.9	91.3	92.0	92.0	•	•	•	•
	T releasing 40 µg/day progesterone	7	20.1	31.5	23.1	26.3	•	•	•	•
	T releasing 65 µg/day progesterone	10	66.0	43.8	39.9	36.9	•	•	•	•
	T releasing 10 µg/day norethisterone	9	54.6	38.4	20.7	50.6	•	•	•	•
	T releasing 2 µg/day d-norgestrel	7	55.8	39.2	25.1	24.2	•	•	•	•

continued to complain of profuse menstruation by the second post-insertion month. This further decreased to 2% by the end of 12 months.

Hefnawi and co-workers (9) compared mean MBL pre- and post-IUD insertion among 19 women using U-coils and among 12 women using progesterone-releasing U-coils. The postinsertion mean MBL for the women with progesterone-releasing U-coils was at least half that of the women with the plain device. In addition, the mean MBLs for the second and third post insertion cycles were lower than the mean MBL in the cycle before insertion.

The preliminary results from a study (30) which compared pre- and postinsertion MBL for the Cu-T and the Progestasert showed about a 50% increase in MBL for 18 Cu-T users after 3, 6 and 12 months of use. For the 18 Progestasert users, the mean MBL declined almost 40% at similar intervals of use.

Studies which have evaluated the patient's perception of her menstrual flow also have documented a decline in complaints of heavy menstrual flow after Progestasert insertion.

Among 169 women who rated their own menstrual flow before and after insertion of Progestasert devices, 14.2% considered their preinsertion flow to be heavy compared to 4.9% after six months of IUD use. At the same time, reports of light flow increased from 15.4% to 35.2% (32).

The Progestasert also may alleviate symptoms of dysmenorrhea. Mild to severe dysmenorrhea reported prior to Progestasert insertion by 56.8% of 169 women decreased after insertion to 43.2% at six months and further to 29.5% at 12 months. The observation of severe dysmenorrhea declined progressively with each month after Progestasert insertion among 253 women who complained of this condition prior to insertion (20).

Duration of Menstrual Blood Loss

While the IUD does not prolong the length of the menstrual cycle (i.e., the interval between the onset of two menstrual periods), it frequently increases the duration of menstrual flow. This statement holds true for all IUDs which have been studied, regardless of their effect on MBL. The exact mechanisms responsible for the increased duration of menstrual flow observed with IUDs are unknown.

> A significantly higher proportion of both nulliparas (20%) and multiparas (18%) who used Cu-T IUDs had menses of seven or more days' duration at six months after insertion compared with the preinsertion experience (4.2% nulliparas and 5% multiparas) (17).
> Wan and co-workers (32) noted that 16% of 169 women had a menstrual flow of six or more days before Progestasert insertion compared to 51.9% at six months after insertion.

Occurrence of Intermenstrual Bleeding

To accurately evaluate the occurrence of intermenstrual bleeding, it would be necessary to have women complete diary cards on which the exact days of bleeding were noted. These data then could be used to assess the frequency and duration of intermenstrual bleeding episodes. With the exception of the Progestasert, the relative frequency of this problem has not been adequately documented in the reported literature for currently available IUDs.

> Rowe and co-workers (26) documented an increased frequency of intermenstrual bleeding in the first month after Progestasert insertion compared to the Cu-7 or to an identical IUD that did not release pro-

gesterone. The increase was most pronounced in the first postinsertion period. The difference between the proportions of women who noted intermenstrual bleeding with a Progestasert or with the other IUDs decreased with time from IUD insertion.

Martinez-Manautou and co-workers (20) reported that the average number of days of intermenstrual bleeding with the Progestasert decreased from about seven days during the first postinsertion cycle to about 1.5 days during the eighth postinsertion cycle.

Pharriss (23) showed that the occurrence of spotting on four or more days during the cycle decreased with increased time from the date of Progestasert insertion among nulliparous and multiparous women.

Mechanisms of IUD-Induced Bleeding

A number of mechanisms have been suggested as possible causes for IUD-induced uterine bleeding. Each of these mechanisms takes into account certain direct physical effects of the device on the endometrium, aside from any pharmacologic effects which may be due to bioactive agents, such as hormones or metals.

IUD distortion and/or displacement are probably the major factors which lead to trauma of the endometrium. Distortion or displacement of the IUD may be due to: 1) disparity between the size and shape of the uterine cavity and the IUD, 2) inaccurate (nonfundal) placement of the device at the time of insertion and 3) increased myometrial contractions induced by the presence of the IUD.

Phatak (24) used hysterography to verify the intrauterine positions of Lippes Loops in 852 women who complained of bleeding, or in whom the IUD strings were not visible. Only 24.1% of the women with normally placed loops complained of bleeding, while this complaint was registered by 60.0% of those with displaced loops and 100.0% of those with distorted loops. Among an asymptomatic group of 100 women, on the other hand, there was no hysterographic evidence of distorted or displaced loops.

A similar correlation between IUD-associated bleeding and a disproportion between the size and shape of the uterine cavity and the IUD based on hysterographic studies was also noted by Kamal and co-workers (11).

There is some evidence to suggest that the traumatic effect of the IUD on the endometrium may contribute to an increased menstrual blood loss via an effect on the blood clotting mechanisms. Rybo (27) reported an increased fibrinolytic activity of the endometrium just before the onset of menstruation. This reached a maximum on the first day of the menstrual period. In addition, he noted a higher concentration of endometrial plasminogen activators in women with menorrhagia than in those who had normal menstrual blood loss. The observations of Rybo (27) have led other investigators to evaluate the effects of the IUD on endometrial fibrinolytic activity.

Larrsson and co-workers (15) observed increased endometrial fibrinolytic activity in 10 of 15 women who used Cu-T or Cu-7 IUDs for at least three months, compared to preinsertion levels.

Kasonde and Bonnar (13) studied the concentration of endometrial plasminogen activators before and after the insertion of a variety of IUDs. An increase in the concentration of plasminogen activators was noted in 16 of the 20 patients. In 2 patients, the observed decrease in concentration may have been related to the different phases of the menstrual cycle during which the pre- and postinsertion endometrial biopsy specimens were obtained.

Bonnar and co-workers (2) evaluated the fibrinolytic activity around a variety of IUDs (Saf-T-Coil, Lippes Loop, Dalkon Shield, Cu-7) removed from 56 women who complained of excessive bleeding and from 24 women who did not complain of excessive bleeding but who wanted to become pregnant. There was a significantly higher ($p < 0.01$) fibrinolytic activity surrounding the IUDs removed from patients for bleeding-related problems.

Anderson and co-workers (1) suggested that IUD-induced menorrhagia may be related to increased endometrial concentrations of prostaglandin E, as well as to increased fibrinolytic activity. In a study of six patients with menorrhagia (including one user of the Cu-7), treatment with flufenamic acid and mefenamic acid (prostaglandin synthetase inhibitors) resulted in a 50% reduction in menstrual blood loss.

Further evidence to support the hypothesis that increased plasminogen activation is a cause of the bleeding irregularities associated with IUD use comes from studies which evaluate the use of antifibrinolytic agents, such as tranexamic acid (AMCA), epsilon aminocaproic acid (EACA) and Trasylol (a naturally occurring pancreatic trypsin inhibitor).

Nilsson and Rybo (22) and Callender and co-workers (3) have reported that orally administered AMCA is effective in the treatment of menorrhagia.

Westrom and Bengtsson (33), in a double-blind study, administered oral AMCA (1.5 gm q.i.d.) to 34 women and a placebo to 31 women during menstrual bleeding after the insertion of Lippes Loops C (58 women), Lippes Loop B (1 woman) and Saf-T-Coils 33S (6 women). In the AMCA-treated group, the mean MBL in the first three post-IUD menstrual cycles was not significantly different from that in the pre-IUD cycles (39.8 ml versus 35.7 ml). In contrast,

the corresponding values among placebo-treated
women were 65.4 ml and 35.8 ml, respectively.

MacMath (18) reported that orally administered
AMCA (3.0 gm q.i.d.) was therapeutically effective
based on the subjective reports of 20 women who
were using Saf-T-Coils and who complained of increased menstrual blood loss.

Kasonde and Bonnar (12) have reported that
orally administered EACA (3.0 gm q.i.d.) also is effective in reducing menstrual blood loss. Among a
group of 56 Lippes Loop D users, 28 were administered EACA during menstruation, and 28 served as
controls. The mean blood loss among the treated
women did not significantly increase after IUD insertion. In the control group, on the other hand, the
mean preinsertion blood loss almost tripled during
the first cycle following IUD insertion, from a mean
of 42.7 ml to a mean of 121.1 ml, but gradually declined to a level about twice that of normal (81.6
ml) by the eighth postinsertion cycle. EACA was not
administered at all during the fifth and seventh cycles. The mean menstrual blood loss for these two
cycles was similar for both the treatment and the control groups. In addition, EACA administration also
appeared to reduce the frequency of intermenstrual
spotting and the severity of menorrhagia in patients
experiencing these symptoms.

Tauber and co-workers (31) evaluated the intrauterine instillation of AMCA and Trasylol in 64 patients who complained of spotting. Both AMCA and
Trasylol reduced the duration of the menstrual flow
by about 50%. These agents also were effective in
stopping intermenstrual bleeding. All women were
using copper-bearing IUDs.

Although the oral or intrauterine administration
of antifibrinolytic agents such as AMCA and Trasylol are effective in reducing MBL and the occurrence
of intermenstrual bleeding, neither can be consid-

ered as a practical therapeutic measure for most patients. Even so, the demonstrated effectiveness of AMCA and Trasylol in the treatment of IUD-induced menorrhagia suggests that IUD acceptability might be enhanced if these agents could be slowly released from the IUD throughout the menstrual cycle.

> Ragab and Thomas (25) evaluated the effects of a U-coil IUD that released AMCA at an average rate of 4 μg per day. The six-month removal rate for bleeding and/or pain for the AMCA-releasing U-coil was 1.1 per 100 women compared to 9.9 per 100 women for a copper-bearing U-coil. Also, reports of increased menstrual bleeding were more frequent among copper U-coil users than for AMCA U-coil users. Menstrual blood loss was not measured in this study.

Significance and Treatment of Uterine Bleeding

Any increase in the duration and the amount of uterine bleeding can be detrimental to the health of women who are prone to anemia or who have borderline nutritional status.

> Among women using either a Birnberg Bow or Antigon IUD whose menstrual blood loss was in excess of 80 ml, a higher proportion developed iron deficiency anemia (31.8%) than did women whose MBL was less than 80 ml (10.5%) per menstrual period (6).

Aside from the effects of excessive bleeding on the hematapoietic reserve of a given woman, *any* change in bleeding patterns may be unacceptable for psychological or cultural reasons and may result in contraceptive discontinuation.

When abnormal uterine bleeding or spotting persists, whether the problem is duration, amount or pattern of bleeding, close attention should be given to the location of the IUD because a partially expelled or displaced device may be the cause of the bleeding. If this is the case, the IUD should be removed and another one inserted if so desired by the patient.

While vasoconstrictors have been prescribed by some physicians as a means of reducing blood loss, such therapy is not recommended on a sustained basis. Persistent, abnormal bleeding requires definitive diagnosis and treatment, beginning with removal of the IUD. Dependent upon the clinical situation, another type of IUD, such as a progesterone-releasing device, may be inserted. Iron supplementation to treat anemia and replenish bone marrow stores is indicated whenever the diagnosis of iron-deficiency anemia is made.

If abnormal uterine bleeding persists after IUD removal, treatment should be related to the underlying medical condition. Hormonal therapy for dysfunctional uterine bleeding may be reasonable for the teenager or younger woman, but persistent uterine bleeding in older women must be investigated by endometrial curettage. Curettage will have a therapeutic effect for endometrial polyps or simple hyperplasia. More serious conditions, including adenomatous hyperplasia and endometrial carcinoma, certainly can occur in women who use IUDs. These conditions represent rare causes of uterine bleeding, but they must not be overlooked, lest appropriate therapy be delayed or omitted.

Despite their apparent effectiveness in reducing the incidence of IUD-induced menstrual disorders, pharmacologic agents, such as the antifibrinolytic agents AMCA and EACA, and the prostaglandin synthetase inhibitors (mefenamic acid, flufenamic acid and ketoprofera), remain experimental and are not accepted at this time for general use because of their possible major side effects.

Summary

All IUDS, with the exception of progestogen-releasing devices, result in increased menstrual blood loss due to increased duration and/or rate of flow. They also may be associated with the increased occurrence of intermenstrual bleeding or spotting. The mechanisms which result in increased uterine bleeding appear to involve both the IUD's direct traumatic effect on the endometrium and an effect on the fibrinolytic system which may inhibit the clotting/fibrinolysis system *in utero*. There is no evidence to indicate that IUDs cause any systemic or generalized effects on the coagulation system.

Considerable research efforts are being directed toward the development of drug-releasing IUDs which will reduce or eliminate the excess uterine bleeding which accompanies the use of most currently available IUDs. The clinical application of such devices does not appear near at hand. Extensive and large-scale clinical trials will be required to assess the possible adverse effects of such devices (including teratogenicity and carcinogenicity) before they can become available for general use.

The persistence of abnormal uterine bleeding in the presence of an IUD indicates removal of the device. If abnormal bleeding persists after removal, immediate and careful diagnosis and treatment are required.

References

1. Anderson, A. B. M.; Guillebaud, J.; Haynes, P. J.; and Turnbull, A. C. Reduction of menstrual blood loss by prostaglandin-synthetase inhibitors. *Lancet* 1:744, 1976.

2. Bonnar, J.; Kasonde, J. M.; Haddon, M.; Hassanein,

M. K.; and Allington, M. J. Fibrinolytic activity in utero and bleeding complications with intrauterine contraceptive devices. *Br. J. Obstet. Gynaecol.* 83:160, 1976.

3. Callender, S. T.; Warner, G. T.; and Cope, E. Treatment of menorrhagia with tranexamic acid. A double-blind trial. *Br. Med. J.* 4:214, 1970.

4. Gallegos, A. J.; Aznar, R.; Merino, G.; and Guizer, E. Intrauterine devices and menstrual blood loss. A comparative study of eight devices during the first six months of use. *Contraception* 17:153, 1978.

5. Guillebaud, J.; Bonnar, J.; Morehead, J.; and Matthews, A. Menstrual blood loss with intrauterine devices. *Lancet* 1:21, 1976.

6. Guttorm, E. Menstrual bleeding with intrauterine contraceptive devices. *Acta Obstet. Gynecol.* (Scand) 50: 9, 1971.

7. Harrison, R. F. Menorrhagia and intrauterine devices. *Lancet* 1:803, 1976.

8. Hefnawi, F.; Askalani, H.; and Zaki, K. Menstrual blood loss with copper intrauterine devices. *Contraception* 9:133, 1974.

9. Hefnawi, F.; Yacout, M. M.; Hosni, M.; El-Sheika, Z.; and Hassanein, M. Medicated intrauterine devices to improve bleeding events. *Int. J. Gynaecol. Obstet.* 15: 79, 1977.

10. Israel, R.; Shaw, S. T.; and Martin, M. A. Comparative quantitation of menstrual blood loss with the Lippes Loop, Dalkon Shield, and Copper T intrauterine devices. *Contraception* 10:63, 1974.

11. Kamal, I.; Hefnawi, F.; Ghoneim, M.; Talaat, M.; and Abdalla, M. Dimensional and architectural disproportion between the intrauterine device and the uterine

cavity. A cause of bleeding. *Fertil. Steril.* 22:514, 1971.

12. Kasonde, J. M., and Bonnar, J. Aminocaproic acid and menstrual loss in women using intrauterine devices. *Br. Med. J.* 4:17, 1975.

13. Kasonde, J. M., and Bonnar, J. Plasminogen activators in the endometrium of women using intrauterine contraceptive devices. *Br. J. Obstet. Gynaecol.* 83:315, 1976.

14. Larsson, B.; Hamberger, L.; and Rybo, G. Influence of copper intrauterine contraceptive devices (Cu-7 IUD) on the menstrual blood loss. *Acta Obstet. Gynecol.* (Scand) 54:315, 1975.

15. Larsson, B.; Liedholm, P.; Sjoberg, N-O.; and Astedt, B. Increased fibrinolytic activity in the endometrium of patients using copper-IUD. *Contraception* 9:531, 1974.

16. Laufe, L. E.; Gibor, Y.; McClanahan, B. J.; and Wheeler, R. F. Volume and copper concentration of menstrual discharge from women employing Copper-7 and other types of contraceptives. *Adv. Plann. Parent.* 9:39, 1974.

17. Liedholm, P.; Rybo, G.; Sjoberg, N-O.; and Solvell, L. Copper IUD influence on menstrual blood loss and iron deficiency. *Contraception* 12:317, 1975.

18. MacMath, I. F. Antifibrinolytic control of menorrhagia after IUD insertion. *Practitioner* 210:417, 1973.

19. Malmquist, R.; Petersohn, L.; and Bengtsson, L. P. Menstrual bleeding with copper-covered intrauterine contraceptive devices. *Contraception* 9:627, 1974.

20. Martinez-Manautou, J.; Correu-Azcona, S.; and Aznar-Ramos, R. Experience in Mexico with the intrauterine hormone contraceptive system (three years of research). *Ginecol. Obstet. Mex.* 40:61, 1976.

21. Nillson, C. G. Comparative quantification of menstrual blood loss with a d-Norgestrel-releasing IUD and a Nova-T copper device. *Contraception* 15:379, 1977.

22. Nilsson, L., and Rybo, G. Treatment of menorrhagia with an antifibrinolytic agent, tranexamic acid (AMCA). A double blind investigation. *Acta Obstet. Gynecol.* (Scand) 46:572, 1967.

23. Pharriss, B. B. Clinical experience with the intrauterine progesterone contraceptive system. *J. Reprod. Med.* 20:155, 1978.

24. Phatak, L. V. Intrauterine distortion and displacement of an IUD. *Indian J. Med. Res.* 56:89, 1969.

25. Ragab, M. I., and Thomas, M. N. The use of tranexamic acid (AMCA) in IUDs as an anti-bleeding agent. *Int. J. Gynaecol. Obstet.* 14:137, 1976.

26. Rowe, P. J.; Koetsawang, S.; Pizarro, E.; and Diethelm, M. P. Comparative bleeding patterns of a progesterone-releasing IUD. In *Analysis of intrauterine contraception*, eds. F. Hefnawi and S. J. Segal. New York: American Elsevier Publishing Co., Inc., 1975.

27. Rybo, G. Plasminogen activators in the endometrium. II. Clinical aspects. *Acta Obstet. Gynecol.* (Scand) 45: 429, 1966.

28. Rybo, G. Menstrual blood loss in relation to parity and menstrual pattern. *Acta Obstet. Gynecol.* (Scand) 45: 25, 1966 (Suppl 7).

29. Rybo, G. Menstrual blood loss associated with intrauterine contraception with copper and progesterone. Abstract in *VIII world congress of gynecology and obstetrics*. Amsterdam: Excerpta Medica, International Congress Series 396, 1976.

30. Rybo, G. The IUD and endometrial bleeding. *J. Reprod. Med.* 20:175, 1978.

31. Tauber, P. F.; Wolf, A. S.; Herting, W.; and Zaneveld, L. J. D. Hemorrhage induced by intrauterine devices: control by local proteinase inhibition. *Fertil. Steril.* 28:1375, 1977.

32. Wan, L. S.; Hsu, Y-C.; Ganguly, M.; and Bigelow, B. Effects of the Progestasert on the menstrual pattern, ovarian steroids and endometrium. *Contraception* 16:417, 1977.

33. Westrom, L., and Bengtsson, L. P. Effect of tranexamic acid (AMCA) in menorrhagia with intrauterine contraceptive devices. A double blind study. *J. Reprod. Med.* 5:154, 1970.

34. World Health Organization. *Expanded program of research, development, and research training in human reproduction.* Fifth Annual Report, November, 1976.

Chapter 6

Cervical and uterine pathology

Background

In the 1950s, Oppenheimer and co-workers (16,17)
were the first to demonstrate that strips of various
plastics and metals were capable of producing neo-
plasms when embedded subcutaneously in rodents.
Subsequent studies by Corfman and Richart (5) confirmed these observations and raised concern about
the possible carcinogenic potential of IUDs.

Corfman and Richart (5) implanted both polyethylene and stainless steel IUDs in Wistar rats to evaluate
the carcogenic potential of these components. Polyethylene is used in the manufacture of Lippes Loops
and stainless steel in a component of the Hall-Stone
Ring. Seven (7%) of the 105 animals with stainless
steel IUDs developed malignant tumors (six epidermoid carcinomas and one sarcoma). The first malignancy was discovered 14 months after the device
was implanted. Among the 102 animals with polyethylene IUDs, six (5.9%) developed malignant uterine tumors (five epidermoid carcinomas and one
sarcoma). In this latter group, the first malignant
tumor was discovered 20 months after implantation.
A control group of 406 rats without IUDs was observed over the same time, and four developed uterine tumors (one adenocarcinoma and three sar-
comas).

It has not yet been established whether the reports on the carcinogenic potential in Wistar rats of various materials used in the manufacture of IUDs relates to the carcinogenic potential of these components when inserted into the human uterus. The findings of Corfman and Richart (5) suggest that any possible association between the IUD and the development of uterine malignancies in the human may not become evident until the IUD has been in use for a prolonged period.

A number of studies have been conducted in humans to assess the possible association between IUD use and uterine cancer. The duration of follow-up for women in most of these studies, however, is less than ten years, and this may not be adequate time to assess any significant increase in the occurrence of uterine or cervical premalignant or malignant changes.

The Papanicolaou-stained smear has been the basis for the evaluation of neoplastic changes in the uterine cervix. The ease with which smears can be obtained and evaluated facilitates the routine screening of large numbers of IUD users for possible neoplastic changes. Papanicolaou smears are often included as part of the routine examination prior to IUD insertion and at yearly follow-up examinations. There is no simple clinical screening procedure for endometrial cancer, so it is not surprising that most cytological follow-up studies of IUD users have focused on the evaluation of the incidence and prevalence of cervical neoplasia rather than on endometrial changes.

Cervical Neoplasia

The reports of Ayre (3) and Pincus and Garcia (18) have been interpreted by some to indicate that the IUD user is at an increased risk of cervical neoplasia.

Table 6.1 The probability of progressing from dysplasia to
carcinoma in situ among IUD users and nonusers.

Days from Study Entry	Cumulative Probability	
	IUD Users	Nonusers
0–90	0.	0.
91–180	0.	0.01
181–360	0.06	0.08
361–540	0.14	0.19
541–720	0.26	0.29
721–900	0.26	0.29

SOURCE: Richart, R. M., and Barron, B. A. (19).

Ayre (3) reported on five women who had a Margulies Spiral inserted. Two of the women with previously normal cervical cytology exhibited cervical changes which rapidly progressed to dysplasia. The other three women had pre-existing mild dysplasia; epithelial changes suggestive of progressing dysplasia were observed only a short period after IUD insertion. Pincus and Garcia (18) reported a rate of suspicious smears (Class III or above) of 5.4% among 500 IUD users. The corresponding rate among a comparable group of women prior to their use of contraception was about 3%.

Richart and Barron (19) compared the rates of progression using the life table method, from dysplasia to carcinoma in situ for 114 IUD users (Birnberg Bow, Lippes Loop, Margulies Spiral, Hall-Stone Ring) and for women who did not use IUDs. All women had a cytologic diagnosis of dysplasia and were followed with only cytologic and colpomicroscopic evaluations. Biopsies or other surgical procedures were not performed unless the lesion progressed to carcinoma in situ or invasive carcinoma. In this study of the natural progression of dysplastic changes, the probability that the lesion would progress from dysplasia to carcinoma in situ was not significantly different for IUD users and nonusers (Table 6.1).

Table 6.2 summarizes the findings from studies which have evaluated the incidence and/or prevalence of cervical neoplasia for women who use various types of IUDs. These studies were selected because they also give the prevalence rates of cervical neoplasia for women who do not use an IUD. The studies cited do not provide any evidence to indicate that IUD users are at a higher risk of cervical neoplasia than are other groups of women. The two groups of women in these studies (IUD users and nonusers) were not, however, necessarily similar with respect to those factors that have been associated with an increased risk of cervical neoplasia (e.g., age, parity, socioeconomic status, age at first coitus). As indicated in Table 6.2, the groups of women who did not use IUDs were not, for the most part, comparable to the IUD user groups. The two groups differed in their ages and parity distributions. In some studies, the dysplasia rates for the nonuser group were prevalence rates (i.e., the percentage of nonusers with dysplasia at one point in time). IUD users were usually followed over time with repeated cytological evaluations; therefore, the calculated dysplasia rate represents a combined incidence and prevalence rate, or an incidence rate, if all women were cytogically normal at the time of IUD insertion. Thus, the calculated dysplasia rates are not comparable for the IUD user and the nonuser groups.

Studies which have reported on cervical neoplasia rates but which have not included any type of control group cannot be used to assess whether or not IUD users are at an increased risk of developing premalignant or malignant cervical lesions. An appropriate comparison group of women who are followed-up is needed to make this assessment.

The available evidence does not indicate a higher risk of cervical neoplasia for IUD users than for nonusers, or for users of different types of IUDs (nonmedicated, copper-bearing or progesterone-releas-

ing). Nor is there evidence at present to suggest that
an IUD in situ will contribute to a more rapid progression of dysplasia to carcinoma in situ or to invasive cancer.

> The study of Richart and Barron (19) referred to earli-
> er showed that the life-table rates of progression from
> dysplasia to carcinoma in situ were not significantly
> different for IUD users and nonusers (Table 6.1).
> Wahi and co-workers (24) reported on 128 wom-
> en who had Lippes Loops inserted and who were
> followed for up to three years. All women had cer-
> vical dysplasia at the time of IUD insertion (60 mild,
> 65 moderate, 3 severe). During the study, the dys-
> plasia progressed to a higher grade for 13.3% of the
> women, to a lower grade or to normal in 30.5% and
> showed no change in 56.2%. In no case did a dys-
> plastic lesion progress to carcinoma in situ or to in-
> vasive cancer.
> Aikat and Aikat (2) followed 14 women who had
> dysplasia prior to insertion of Lippes Loops. All the
> women had negative smears within one year of the
> IUD insertion.

The presence of dysplasia is not an absolute
contraindication to the insertion of an IUD, even
though some physicians may prefer not to insert a
device until the dysplasia has been treated. Women
with cervical neoplasia should be treated promptly;
the type of treatment will depend on the extent and
type of lesion. Removal of the IUD is not required for
women who have dysplastic lesions and who will be
treated expectantly or with electrocautery, cryocau-
tery or punch biopsies, although removal is often
performed to facilitate ease of treatment. It is important to prevent pregnancy for these women until
treatment has been completed. If the IUD is removed,
other suitable contraceptive measures must be of-
fered. The occurrence of pregnancy with an IUD in

Table 6.2 Rates of cervical neoplasia.

Reference Number	Contraceptive Method	Number of Subjects	Study Findings			Comments
			Percentage with smears Class III or above			
18	Vaginal	208	7.2			Average duration of contraceptive use (years): Vaginal, 1.3; Orals, 1.6–3.4; IUD, 1.1
	Orals					
	Enovid	580	2.6			
	Ovulen	188	2.1			
	Orthonovum	105	2.9			
	IUD (type not stated)	500	5.4			
			Dysplasia (%)	Carcinoma in situ (%)	Carcinoma (%)	
10	IUD (mostly Yusei rings)	1,333	6.4	0.0	0.0	Nonusers were older than IUD users. Some IUD users were followed for over 10 years; 75% followed for over 5 years. Dysplasia rate was not related to duration of IUD use.
	Not IUD Users	7,226	7.1	0.2	0.01	

		CIN$_1$	CIN$_2$	CIN$_3$	Carcinoma	
					(Rates per 1,000 woman-years)	
6	Long-acting progestogens (medroxyprogesterone acetate, chlormadinone acetate)	2,684	0.42	0.28	0.42	0.14	Users of long-acting progestogens were older and of higher parity than IUD users.
	IUD—Lippes Loop	2,409	0.91	0.61	0.00	0.30	Prevalence rates of neoplasia at admission to the study: Progestogen group, 1.3%; IUD group, 0.7%; 1 case of carcinoma in each group.
12	IUD (Cu-T, Cu-7)	490	Dysplasia rates (%) at 6, 12, 18 and 24 months postinsertion: 2.5, 5.5, 2.7 and 1.4.				Prevalence of dysplasia in general population: 2.4%.
			Dysplasia rate (%)				
8	IUD (Cu-T, Cu-7)	229	4.4				A single smear was performed for nonuser group. IUD users were followed for up to 8 years with repeat smears. Both groups similar with respect to age and parity. Results of preinsertion smears not available for IUD group.
	Not IUD Users	296	4.7				

situ in association with cervical neoplasia presents an added complication to both the physician and the patient.

Uterine Cancer

Uterine cancer occurs most frequently in women over the age of 50, with only about 4% of uterine cancers occurring before the age of 40 (7). The incidence of uterine cancer is about 0.5% for women of reproductive age. Most studies which have histologically evaluated endometrial changes following the insertion of an IUD have been limited by the short duration of follow-up and the relatively small numbers of subjects. It is unlikely that studies which involve a few hundred IUD users are sufficiently large enough to detect any significant increase in the incidence of uterine cancer.

Numerous studies (1,4,9,11,13,15,20,22,23,25) have shown that histologic alterations in the endometrium do occur following the insertion of an IUD. However, most of these changes are representative of a mild inflammatory reaction (chronic endometritis) and probably represent a foreign body reaction to the IUD. Except for the study of Hata and co-workers (10) in 1969, the endometrial histology of IUD users was not compared to that of nonusers.

> Hata and co-workers (10) compared the endometrial histology of 495 Yusei ring users to that of 69 women who did not use IUDs. Inflammatory changes were more frequent among the IUD users; otherwise, there were no significant differences between the histology of the two groups. There was no apparent association between the histologic appearance of the endometrium and the duration of IUD use.

Most investigations have evaluated the histologic changes of the endometrium by random endometrial biopsies. The following study was undertaken specifically to examine the endometrium in proximity to the IUD.

> Abrams and Spritzer (1) evaluated the endometrium adherent to IUDs (modification of the Gräfenberg Ring) electively removed from 50 women who had used them for at least one year. The endometrium was compared with routine endometrial aspirates from 500 premenopausal women. The specimens from both groups were found to be morphologically similar.

Studies which have evaluated the histology of the endometrium have not provided any evidence to suggest that the IUD has a carcinogenic potential. These studies have in effect only evaluated the short-term effects of the IUD on the endometrium. Cases of endometrial hyperplasia have been occasionally reported among IUD users, but its frequency of occurrence is estimated to be less than 0.5%.

Summary

The existing literature does not demonstrate an association between IUD use and an increased risk of cervical or endometrial neoplasia, either benign or malignant. It may, however, be difficult or impossible to detect such an association because of the practical limitations of conducting large scale studies with long term follow up that may extend over decades. The discovery of cervical dysplasia, endometrial hyperplasia or frank cancer of the uterine cervix or corpus requires the same diagnostic evaluation and treatment for the IUD user as for the woman who does not use an IUD.

References

1. Abrams, R. Y., and Spritzer, T. Endometrial cytology in patients using intrauterine contraceptive devices. *Acta Cytol.* 10:240, 1966.

2. Aikat, M., and Aikat, B. K. Long term effect of Lippes Loop on cervical epithelium and endometrium. *Ind. J. Med. Res.* 61:1313, 1973.

3. Ayre, J. E. Human precarcinogenic cell manifestations associated with polyethylene contraceptive device. *Ind. Med. Surg.* 34:393, 1965.

4. Bonney, W. A.; Glasser, S. R.; Clewe, T. H.; Noyes, R. W.; and Cooper, C. L. Endometrial response to the intrauterine device. *Am. J. Obstet. Gynecol.* 96:101, 1966.

5. Corfman, P. A., and Richart, R. M. Uterine epidermoid carcinoma induced in rats by plastic and stainless steel intra-uterine devices. *Excerpta Medica International Congress Series* No. 156:89, 1968.

6. Dabancens, A.; Prado, R.; Larraguibel, R.; and Zanartu, J. Intraepithelial cervical neoplasia in women using intrauterine devices and long-acting progestogens as contraceptives. *Am. J. Obstet. Gynecol.* 19:1052, 1974.

7. Disaia, P. J.; Morrow, C. P.; and Townsend, D. E. *Synopsis of Gynecologic Onocology.* New York: John Wiley and Sons, 1975.

8. Engineer, A. D., and Misra, J. S. Cytological studies in women using intrauterine contraception. *Ind. J. Med. Res.* 64:1255, 1976.

9. Fornasi, M. L. Cellular changes in the glandular epithelium of patients using IUCD—a source of cytologic error. *Acta Cytol.* 18:341, 1974.

10. Hata, Y; Ishihama, A.; Kudo, N.; Nakamura, Y.; Miyai,

T.; Makino, T.; and Kagabu, T. The effect of long-term use of intrauterine devices. *Int. J. Fertil.* 14:241, 1969.

11. Israel, R., and Davis, H. J. Effect of intrauterine contraceptive devices on the endometrium. *JAMA* 195:765, 1966.

12. Luthra, U. K.; Mitra, A. B.; Bhinder, G.; Bhatnagar, P.; and Saxena, N. C. Surveillance for carcinogenesis in women using Cu-IUD for contraception. *Ind. J. Med. Res.* 63:1787, 1975.

13. Moyer, D. L., and Mishell, D. R. Reactions of human endometrium to the intrauterine foreign body. II. Long-term effects on the endometrial histology and cytology. *Am. J. Obstet. Gynecol.* 111:66, 1971.

14. Ober, W. B.; Sobrero, A. J.; and de Chabon, A. B. Endometrial findings after insertion of stainless steel spring IUD. *Obstet. Gynecol.* 36:62, 1970.

15. Ober, W. B.; Sobrero, A. J.; de Chabon, A. B.; and Goodman, J. Polyethylene intrauterine contraceptive device. Endometrial changes following long-term use. *JAMA* 212:765, 1970.

16. Oppenheimer, B. S.; Oppenheimer, E. T.; Stout, A. P.; and Danishefsky, L. Malignant tumors resulting from embedding plastics in rodents. *Science* 116:305, 1953.

17. Oppenheimer, B. S.; Oppenheimer, E. T.; Danishefsky, L.; and Stout, A. P. Carcinogenic effects of metals in rodents. *Cancer Res.* 16:349, 1956.

18. Pincus, G., and Garcia, C.-R. Studies on vaginal, cervical and uterine histology. *Metabolism* 14:344, 1965.

19. Richart, R. M., and Barron, B. A. The intrauterine device and cervical neoplasia. A prospective study of patients with cervical dysplasia. *JAMA* 199:817, 1967.

20. Sammour, M. B.; Iskander, S. G.; and Rifai, S. F. Combined histologic and cytologic study of intrauterine contraception. *Am. J. Obstet. Gynecol.* 98:946, 1967.

21. Shahani, S. M.; Dandekas, P. V.; and Chikhlikas, A. R. Intrauterine devices: effectiveness and changes in the genital tract. *Excerpta Medica International Congress Series* No. 133:1138, 1967.

22. Shahani, S. M., and Kothari, U. R. Effect of long-term insertion of I.U.D. on human endometrium. *J. Obstet. Gynaecol.* (India) XXIII:235, 1973.

23. Sujan-Tejuja, S.; Virick, R. K.; and Malkani, P. K. Uterine histopathology in the presence of intra-uterine devices. *Excerpta Medica International Congress Series* No. 86:172, 1964.

24. Wahi, P. N.; Lahiri, V. L.; Mali, S.; and Luthra, U. K. Study of cervical epithelial changes in women using Lippes' Loop. *Ind. J. Med. Res.* 56:294, 1968.

25. Willson, J. R.; Ledger, W. J.; and Andros, G. J. The effects of the intrauterine device on the histologic pattern of the endometrium. *Am. J. Obstet. Gynecol.* 93:802, 1966.

Chapter 7

Intrauterine pregnancy

Introduction

The IUD is intended to prevent pregnancy; nevertheless, pregnancies have occurred with IUDs in situ. In most instances, the reasons for this method failure are unknown.

Kamal and co-workers (28) have suggested that uterine abnormalities and a disproportion between the size or shape of the uterine cavity and the IUD lead to displacement or disorientation of the IUD and subsequent pregnancy. If the effect of the IUD is local and related to the area of endometrial contact, then the displaced IUD leaves part of the uterus unprotected and thereby allows conception to occur.

Gawad and co-workers (18) studied women who became pregnant with the IUD (Lippes Loop) in situ, and found that the device had provoked a lesser degree of intrauterine cellular reaction in terms of the number of polymorphonuclear cells, macrophages, lymphocytes and endometrial cells obtained by uterine flushing in these women than it had in women who did not become pregnant.

The studies by Kamal and co-workers (28) and Gawad and co-workers (18) suggest means by which contraceptive failure may occur. There is, however, little hope that an IUD with a zero failure rate and acceptable rates of expulsion and removal for pain

and bleeding will be developed until the mechanisms of IUD action are more clearly understood. It
is possible to develop an IUD with a near zero pregnancy rate, but such IUDs, the Spring Coil (41), for
example, are associated with high rates of removal
for pain and bleeding. Moreover, the Spring Coil is
difficult to insert and its expulsion is highly probable if the insertion is incorrect.

The outcome of those pregnancies which occur
with IUDs in situ are of concern to physicians and
patients. Some women will elect to have their pregnancies terminated by abortion; others will elect to
carry their pregnancies to term. It is important that
the woman who wishes to continue her pregnancy
be advised of her potential for a term pregnancy and
of the possible risks to the fetus caused by the presence of the IUD at the time of conception.

Outcome of Pregnancy

The outcome of pregnancies which occur with IUDs
in situ are less favorable than the outcome of pregnancies which occur because other contraceptive
methods have failed. There is a higher precentage of
both ectopic pregnancies (see Chapter 8) and spontaneous abortion among women who become pregnant due to the method failure of an IUD.

> Vessey and co-workers (50) reported that the rate of
> spontaneous abortion was about three times higher
> (55.7%) among women with IUD failures (Lippes
> Loop, Saf-T-Coil, M, Dalkon Shield, Cu-7 and others)
> than it was among women who experienced failures
> with other contraceptive methods (17.1%) (Table
> 7.1).

Any evaluation of the outcome of pregnancies
conceived with IUDs in situ must make a distinction
between those pregnancies where the IUDs were left

Table 7.1 Outcomes of pregnancies among parous women according to the failed contraceptive method.

Pregnancy Outcome	Method of Contraception			
	IUD N = 115 (%)	Orals N = 22 (%)	Diaphragm N = 166 (%)	Others/None N = 122 (%)
Live birth	33.9	86.4	80.1	80.4
Stillbirth	1.7	0.0	1.8	1.6
Spontaneous abortion	55.7	13.6	18.1	16.4
Ectopic	8.7	0.0	0.0	1.6

SOURCE: Vessey et al. (50).

in place and those where the devices were removed or expelled before termination of the pregnancies. In either instance, the outcome of pregnancies resulting from IUD failure is less favorable than the outcome of pregnancies from failures of other contraceptive methods. Table 7.2 presents the results of three studies which compared the outcome of pregnancies where IUDs were left in situ to the outcome of pregnancies where the IUDs were expelled or removed before termination of the pregnancies. Although spontaneous abortion may occur if the IUD is left in situ, there is about a 2.3-fold increased risk of spontaneous abortion if the IUD is not removed or expelled. The differences among the spontaneous abortion rates in Table 7.2 may be due to a number of factors, including the duration of the various pregnancies and the location of the IUD when the devices were removed or expelled, the type of IUD and the special reasons for its removal. In Alvior's (4) study, the criteria for IUD removal required that the IUD string was visible at the cervical os, pregnancy had not advanced beyond the first trimester and no undue resistance was evident during the first attempt at removal. The criteria for IUD removal were not stated by Tatum and co-workers (47) or by Last (30).

The location of the IUD at the time of conception also may have an effect on the outcome of the pregnancy. If the IUD is displaced into the lower

Table 7.2 Outcome of pregnancies conceived with the IUD in
situ.

Reference Number	IUD	IUD Left In Situ			
		Number of Pregnancies	LB (%)	SB (%)	SA (%)
4	Lippes Loop	120	51.7	0.0	48.3
30	Lippes Loop	16	25.0	0.0	75.0
47	Cu-T	157	44.0	1.9	54.1
Total		293	46.1	1.0	52.9
Reference Number	IUD	IUD Removed or Expelled after Conception			
		Number of Pregnancies	LB (%)	SB (%)	SA (%)
4	Lippes Loop	81	69.2	1.2	29.6
30	Lippes Loop	5	100.0	0.0	0.0
47	Cu-T	118	78.8	0.9	20.3
Total		204	75.5	1.0	23.5

NOTE: LB = live birth, SB = stillbirth, SA = spontaneous abortion.

uterine segment or partially expelled into the cervix,
then removal or nonremoval may have a lesser effect on the pregnancy than if the IUD were properly
positioned.

Removal of the IUD by gentle traction on its
strings is potentially less traumatic to the pregnancy
than probing the uterus to locate and remove the
IUD. If the IUD strings are not visible at the cervical
os and the woman wishes to carry her pregnancy to
term, the uterus should not be probed to locate the
IUD. In some cases, the IUD will have been expelled
and probing of the uterus will only increase the
chances of interrupting the pregnancy. The spontaneous abortion rates following removal or expulsion of an IUD (23.5%, Table 7.2) appear to be only
slightly higher than spontaneous abortion rates
among women who do not use IUDs (17.1%, Table
7.1).

Life table rates should be computed to compare
the spontaneous abortion rates for IUD users and
nonusers, as well as for different types of IUDs.
Women who choose to terminate their pregnancies

by induced abortion are at risk of spontaneous abortion only until the time of induced termination. Spontaneous abortion rates in published studies only approximate the true risk of spontaneous abortion because they are calculated as a percentage of known pregnancy outcomes and exclude those women who underwent an induced abortion. Moreover, published spontaneous abortion rates do not provide any indication of the risks of a spontaneous abortion as it relates to gestational age, regardless of whether or not the IUD was removed. Nevertheless, the literature contains many useful reports of the spontaneous abortion rates for different types of IUDs, and these are presented in Table 7.3 as a reference for the reader. Most reports cited in this table do not provide the information necessary to categorize the spontaneous abortion rates according to whether or not the IUD was removed, expelled or left in situ after conception.

The data in Table 7.3 show a higher rate of spontaneous abortion for the Dalkon Shield than for the

Table 7.3 Rate and number of spontaneous abortions for different types of IUDs.

IUD	Rate (%)	Number of Spontaneous Abortions	Reference Number
Lippes Loop	43.4	23	20
(all sizes)	40.8	82	4
	39.7	23	16
Saf-T-Coil	14.7	5	16
Dalkon Shield	77.1	27	33
	58.1	18	1
	61.0	100	16
Cu-T	40.2	113	47
	25.0	1	16
Cu-7	31.7	53	45
	41.5	27	16
Progestasert	48.3	14	5

Table 7.4 *Number of spontaneous abortions and number and
rate of septic spontaneous abortions for different IUDs.*

Reference Number		Spontaneous Abortions (No.)	Septic Abortions	
			Number	Rate (%)
20	Lippes Loop	23	4	17.4
45	Cu-7	53	0	0.0
1	Dalkon Shield	18	1	5.6
55	Dalkon Shield	4	0	0.0
	Lippes Loop ⎫ Saf-T-Coil ⎬ Unknown ⎭	54	4	7.4
47	Cu-T	113	2	1.8
16	Dalkon Shield	100	2	2.0

other IUDs cited. This finding must be interpreted
with care in view of the small number of reports on
spontaneous abortion rates. Possible reasons for the
increased spontaneous abortion rate associated with
the Dalkon Shield include various design features
unique to this device. The protrusions on the periph-
ery of the Dalkon Shield may cause trauma to the
fetal membranes which lead to spontaneous abortion, or they may impinge on the endometrium and
contribute to an increased susceptibility to infection
which may result in fetal loss. In addition, it has
been hypothesized that the tail of the Dalkon Shield
provides a nidus for infection which may result in
spontaneous abortion (46). If this were so, such infections could be expected to become clinically evident in many pregnancies which occur with the Dalkon Shield in situ. The available data do not support
this supposition. When the septic spontaneous abortion rate is calculated as a percentage of spontaneous
abortions, the Dalkon Shield does not appear to be
associated with a higher septic spontaneous abortion
rate than other IUDs (Table 7.4). This conclusion
must be considered tentative because the criteria for
the diagnosis of septic abortion were not always stated in the reports in Table 7.4, and because of the

relatively few reports from which septic spontaneous abortion rates could be calculated.

Septic Complications of Pregnancy

A mail survey of 8,506 physicians was conducted in
1967 in the United States, Canada and Puerto Rico to
determine the extent of critical illness and death
which resulted from PID or complications of uterine
perforation in association with the use of IUDs. Ten
deaths were reported (42), two of which resulted
from amniotic fluid embolism following second trimester deliveries. Uterine perforations were revealed at autopsy in both cases. In a third case, the
tentative diagnosis of septic abortion was not confirmed at autopsy. Scott (42) also reported 369 cases
of infection, some of which were associated with
pregnancy. Although Scott's report (42) did not estimate the risks of serious complications associated
with IUD use, it did emphasize that potentially serious and sometimes fatal complications do occur in
both gravid and nongravid women.

Christian (13) reported subsequently on five
midtrimester deaths and seven cases of severe sepsis
associated with in situ IUDs in midtrimester pregnancies. Four of the five deaths and six of the seven
cases of severe sepsis occurred in women using Dalkon Shields. In the other two cases, Lippes Loops
were used. Christian's report (13) did not provide
any statistical association between IUD use and complicated pregnancies. It did present sufficient evidence to warrant further evaluation of the possible
association between the use of an IUD, the Dalkon
Shield in particular, and complicated pregnancies.

In 1973, the Center for Disease Control (CDC)
conducted a mail survey of physicians in the United
States and Puerto Rico who were most likely to be
involved with intrauterine contraception. The object
of the survey was to determine IUD-related mortality

and morbidity rates severe enough to require hospi-
talizaion. Kahn and Tyler (27) reported two observations from this survey which suggested a higher risk
of complicated pregnancies with the Dalkon Shield
than with other IUDs. Dalkon Shield users evidenced a higher percentage (37.6%) of hospitalizations for complicated pregnancies than did users of
other IUDs (22.2%) (Lippes Loop, Saf-T-Coil and
other known IUDs). This was reflected in a higher
odds ratio of 2.1 (95% confidence limits, 1.8–2.4)
which indicates that the ratio of complicated pregnancies to other diagnoses is about twice as high for
Dalkon Shield users as it is for users of other IUDs.
The study did not indicate whether there was an
increased rate of complicated pregnancies or a decreased rate of complications not related to pregnancy. Kahn and Tyler (27) also observed that about
40% of the IUD users were using the Dalkon Shield
at the time of the survey and that this device accounted for 61.6% of all hospitalizations with a diagnosis of complicated pregnancy. The CDC survey
had a response rate of only 49.4% which prompted
the investigators to obtain a 1% random sample of
the nonrespondents. An analysis of the responses
from the random sampling yielded results similar to
those of the original survey.

In an unpublished report which commented on
the CDC survey, Mosley and co-workers (38) found
that the rate of hospitalization for Dalkon Shield
users was about 4 to 18% higher than it was for users
of other IUDs after adjusting for duration of IUD use.
This difference could be attributed to a higher pregnancy rate for the Dalkon Shield compared to other
IUDs.

The Food and Drug Administration held a meeting in October 1974 to present data relating to the
Dalkon Shield and other IUDs. A total of 219 cases of
complicated pregnancy, including 13 deaths, were
reported for the Dalkon Shield, while 68 cases of

nber of
ths

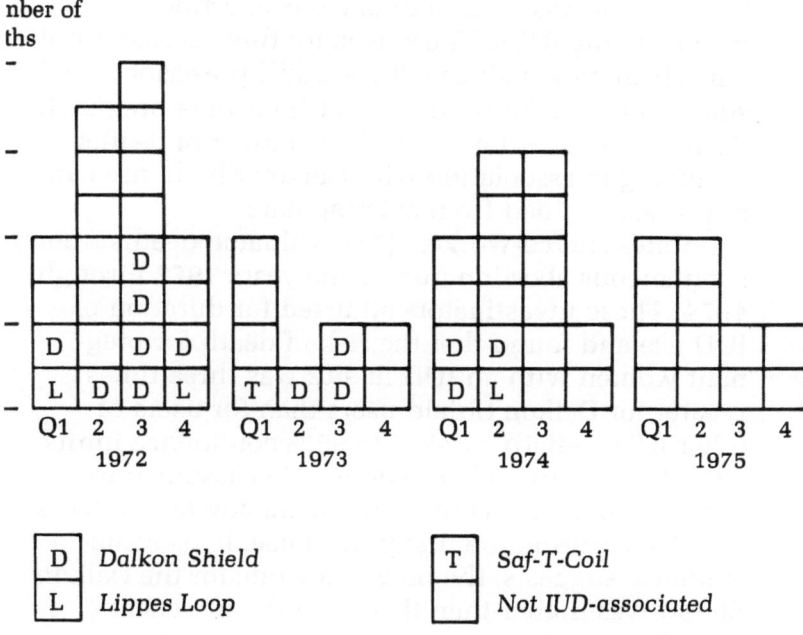

| D | Dalkon Shield | T | Saf-T-Coil |
| L | Lippes Loop | | Not IUD-associated |

SOURCE: Cates et al. (12)

Figure 7.1: Spontaneous abortion deaths in the United States, 1972–1975.

complicated pregnancy, including 7 deaths, were reported for other IUDs (Lippes Loop, Saf-T-Coil, Margulies Spiral, Birnberg Bow, Hall Band).

Reports on the possible association between
septic spontaneous abortion and IUD use have led to
an increased awareness of the risks to the IUD user
who becomes pregnant with an IUD in situ. From
January 1972 to July 1974 in the United States, there
were seventeen reported deaths from spontaneous
abortion associated with an in situ IUD (Dalkon
Shield, 13; Lippes Loop, 3; Saf-T-Coil, 1) (Fig. 7.1).
Cates and co-workers (12) reported no deaths from
spontaneous abortion for women using any type of
IUD from July 1974 to April 1977 in the United
States. Since the publication of this report there have

been two deaths from spontaneous abortion for
women using IUDs. The reason for this decline is not
entirely apparent since IUDs are still prescribed, and
some women who wear them still become pregnant.
Also, the reasons for the higher number of deaths
occurring in association with Dalkon Shield use cannot be ascertained from existing data.

Cates and co-workers (11) evaluated deaths from
spontaneous abortion during the years 1972 through
1974. These investigators adjusted for duration of
IUD use and found that the risk of death for pregnant women with an IUD in situ was three times
greater for Dalkon Shield users than for users of
other IUDs (relative risk, 3.0; 95% confidence limits,
1.04–8.8). Cates and co-workers (11) assumed for
purposes of analysis that the pregnancy rate of IUDs
was 2.4% during the first year of use. If, as some
evidence suggests, the pregnancy rate for the Dalkon
Shield was higher than this, then the net effect
would be a reduction in the magnitude of the risk
of death. Whether or not this risk would remain significantly higher for the Dalkon Shield compared to
other IUDs depends on the assumed pregnancy rates,
as well as on the number of women using each type
of IUD and on the duration of use.

Septic complications of pregnancy associated
with IUD use have been reported for most IUDs (2,3,
6,9,10,13,15,17,21,22,25,34,36,37,39,40,43,48,51,52,
54,56). Most of the literature, however, presents
reports which do not establish any association between IUD use, or use of a particular IUD, and the
type of septic complication.

Management of Pregnancies with an
IUD in Situ

The reported cases of septic spontaneous abortion
which occur in association with the Dalkon Shield
and other IUDs have heightened clinical awareness

of the potential seriousness of complications which may result when pregnancy occurs with an IUD in situ. At present, the recommended and accepted clinical practice dictates removal of an IUD whenever pregnancy is diagnosed. Difficulties arise when the IUD strings are not visible or cannot be located in the cervical canal. This may not present a problem for the woman who does not wish to remain pregnant because her pregnancy can be safely terminated by abortion. If the woman wishes to continue her pregnancy to term, attempts should be made to confirm the intrauterine presence of the IUD. Although the use of ultrasound has some advantages for the pregnant woman, this technique has failed some investigators (23,24,26) in their attempts to locate the intrauterine presence of an IUD in pregnant patients.

The woman who wishes to continue her pregnancy to term with an IUD *in utero* presents a dilemma to the physician. Any probing of the uterus may disrupt the pregnancy, but leaving the IUD in situ increases the risk of a spontaneous abortion. The woman who elects to continue her pregnancy with an IUD in situ must be followed closely. Both the physician and the patient should be alert to any symptoms suggesting sepsis or impending abortion. If sepsis occurs or is suspected, immediate antibiotic therapy should be initiated, and the uterus should be evacuated and the IUD removed by the most expedient method. After evacuation, the uterus should be carefully explored to assure that all tissue has been removed. Inadequate evacuation of the uterus may prolong the septic condition and place the patient at risk of additional complications (14,56).

It is mandatory that prompt treatment be provided to the patient who has an IUD in situ and presents with any symptoms of an impending abortion. In many instances, the initial symptoms may not seem to be cause for alarm, but death from sepsis has been reported within 72 hours of the onset of symptoms. Christian (13) has commented that the infection may become generalized prior to or concurrent with the appearance of any localizing signs. Prompt treatment is, therefore, crucial.

Congenital Abnormalities

It does not appear that congenital abnormalities occur more frequently in babies born to women who conceived with an IUD *in utero* (Table 7.5). Since there is also evidence to indicate that the IUD prevents congenital abnormalities, the frequency of occurrence can be expected to be the same as for a noncontracepting population.

It must be recognized that congenital abnormalities may go undetected. Many pregnancies conceived with the IUD *in utero* are terminated either electively or spontaneously before the fetus has developed to an age or size which permits the detection of abnormalities. Even when a terminated pregnancy is sufficiently advanced to permit detection of a congenital abnormality, such abnormalities may go unnoticed unless they are specifically being searched for.

The study of Layde and co-workers (31) is the only one which has specifically evaluated the association between IUD use and congenital abnormalities. In this study, no increased risk of limb reduction deformities was found among the offspring of women who reported they conceived with an IUD in situ, as compared to women who reported they did not have an IUD in situ at conception.

It has been estimated that over 15 million women have used IUDs. If it is assumed that 1% to 3% of these women become pregnant with IUDs in situ, then between 150,000 and 450,000 pregnancies would be expected. If as few as 20% of these women carried their pregnancies to term and 5% of the babies born had congenital abnormalities, then 1,500

Table 7.5 Congenital abnormalities among pregnancies conceived with an IUD in situ.

Reference Number	IUD	Congenital Abnormality	Number of Cases	Rate/100 Pregnancies
8	Birnberg Bow	Microcephalus, fetus papyraceus (twin pregnancy)	1	—
49	Lippes Loop Margulies Spiral Birnberg Bow Steel Ring Other	Phocomelia Meningocele	1 1	} 0.7
42	Saf-T-Coil	Deformed lower extremity	1	—
6	Not stated	Double-headed monster	1	5.3
44	Dalkon Shield Saf-T-Coil Lippes Loop Cu-7 Unknown	Cleft Palate	1	4.3

Table 7.5 (con't)

Reference Number	IUD	Congenital Abnormality	Number of Cases	Rate/100 Pregnancies
7	Grafenberg Ring Dalkon Shield*	} Fibular aplasia and related limb reduction defects	2	—
19	Cu-7	Permanent bald spot on head Bilateral ptosis of eyelid Lipoma on back Congenital dislocation of hip Lumbosacral meningomylocele and bilateral clubfoot	1 1 1 1 1	3.0
32	Not stated	Limb reduction defect	1	—
35	Dalkon Shield	Duplication of urethra	1	—
47	Cu-T	Benign fibroma of vocal cord	1	0.06
31	Not stated	Limb reduction deformity Chromosomal defect Other major defects		

*Patient did not identify the IUD she had used until three months after delivery. It was not ascertained whether the Dalkon Shield was the IUD used or whether it was in situ at conception.

to 4,500 congenital abnormalities would be expected. The congenital abnormalities reported in Table 7.5 represent only a small fraction of this expected number; thus, it seems most unlikely that the IUD causes congenital abnormalities.

Summary

The outcomes of pregnancies conceived with IUDs in situ are less favorable than the outcomes of pregnancies which occur due to the failure of other contraceptive methods. Higher rates for both ectopic pregnancy and spontaneous abortion are associated with the failure of IUDs than with the failure of other contraceptive methods. The risk of spontaneous abortion is about two times greater if the IUD is not removed once pregnancy has been confirmed. The rate of spontaneous abortion appears to be similar for all types of IUDs, except the Dalkon Shield which has a higher rate than other devices. The proportions of septic spontaneous abortions appear to be similar for all IUDs, including the Dalkon Shield.

Women who become pregnant with an IUD in situ should be advised to have their IUDs removed. If, after counseling, a woman wishes to continue her pregnancy with the device in situ, she should be followed closely and advised to report any signs or symptoms of possible infection at once.

No evidence has been reported in the literature to suggest that any type of IUD causes congenital abnormalities.

References

1. A. H. Robins Company, Unpublished data. Richmond, Virginia.

2. Acosta, A. A.; Mabray, C. R.; and Kaufman, R. H. Intra-

uterine pregnancy and coexistent pelvic inflammatory disease. *Obstet. Gynecol.* 37:282, 1971.

3. Agnew, H. W.; and Pritchard, J. A. Abortion and bacterial shock induced with an intrauterine contraceptive device. Report of a case. *Obstet. Gynecol.* 28:332, 1966.

4. Alvior, G. T. Pregnancy outcome with removal of intrauterine device. *Obstet. Gynecol.* 41:894, 1973.

5. Alza Corporation. *The Progestasert.* Intrauterine progesterone contraceptive system release rated 65 μg/day progesterone for one year. Alza Product Information, Palo Alto, California, 1977.

6. Baker, J. W. Serious complications of intrauterine contraceptive devices. *Med. J. Australia* 1:1126, 1969.

7. Barrie, H. Congenital malformation associated with intrauterine contraceptive device. *Br. Med. J.* 1:488, 1976.

8. Beck, P.; Birnbaum, S. J.; and Schlossberg, M. Intrauterine contraceptive device failure associated with anomalous full-term delivery. *N.Y. State J. Med.*, June 15:1766, 1967.

9. Biggerstaff, E. D.; Menutti, M. T.; Yetter, J. F.; and Rogers, R. E. Maternal midtrimester sepsis in association with the intrauterine contraceptive device: early histopathologic findings. *Am. J. Obstet. Gynecol.* 124:207, 1976.

10. Boyd, J. J., and Rawlinson, K. F. Third-trimester uterine sepsis associated with shield-type intrauterine device. *Lancet* 1:813, 1975.

11. Cates, W.; Ory, H. W.; Rochat, R. W.; and Tyler, C. W. The intrauterine device and deaths from spontaneous abortion. *N. Engl. J. Med.* 295:1155, 1976.

12. Cates, W.; Grimes, D. A.; Ory, H. W.; and Tyler, C. W.

Publicity and the public health: the elimination of IUD-related abortion deaths. *Fam. Plann. Perspec.* 9: 138, 1977.

13. Christian, C. D. Maternal deaths associated with an intrauterine device. *Am. J. Obstet. Gynecol.* 119:441, 1974.

14. Christian, C. D. The morbidity and mortality of mid-trimester sepsis associated with IUDs. In *Analysis of intrauterine contraception*, eds. F. Hefnawi and S. J. Segal. New York: American Elsevier Publishing Co., Inc., 1975.

15. Eisinger, S. H. Second-trimester spontaneous abortion, the IUD, and infection. *Am. J. Obstet. Gynecol.* 124: 393, 1976.

16. Family Planning Research Unit. *An enquiry into the data base on the Dalkon Shield*, Memorandum no. 3. Exeter: The Family Planning Research Unit, University of Exeter, 1977.

17. Gabel, G. H., and Dunn, L. J. A possible new hazard of the intrauterine contraceptive device. *Virginia Med. Monthly* 102:20, 1975.

18. Gawad, A. H. A.; Toppozada, H. K.; Sawi, M. D.; Salleh, F.; and Sahwi, S. E. Study of the environment in association with intrauterine contraceptive devices. *Contraception* 16:469, 1977.

19. Guillebaud, J. IUD and congenital malformation. *Br. Med. J.* 1:1016, 1976.

20. Hall, R. E. A Four Year Report on Loop D. *Int. J. Fertil.* 13:309, 1968.

21. Ho, C-Y, and Aterman, K. Infection of the Fetus by candida in a spontaneous abortion. *Am. J. Obstet. Gynecol.* 106:705, 1970.

22. Hurt, W. G. Septic pregnancy associated with Dalkon

Shield intrauterine device. *Obstet Gynecol.* 44:491, 1974.

23. Ianniruberto, A., and Mastroberardino, A. Ultrasonic localization of the Lippes Loop. *Am. J. Obstet. Gynecol.* 114:78, 1972.

24. Janssens, D.; Vrijens, M.; Thiery, M.; and Van Kets, H. Ultrasonic detection, localization and identification of intrauterine contraceptive devices. *Contraception* 8:485, 1973.

25. Jewett, J. F. Chorioamnionitis complicated by an intrauterine device (Committee on Maternal Welfare: Massachusetts Medical Society). *N. Engl. J. Med.* 289: 1251, 1973.

26. Jouppila, P. Location of the missing intrauterine contraceptive device. *Acta Obstet Gynecol.* (Scand) 54:71, 1975.

27. Kahn, H. S., and Tyler, C. W. An association between the Dalkon Shield and complicated pregnancies among women hospitalized for intrauterine contraceptive device-related disorders. *Am. J. Obstet. Gynecol.* 125:83, 1976.

28. Kamal, I.; Ghoneim, M.; Talaat, M.; Abdalla, M.; Eid, M.; and Rawai, E. Pregnancies in the presence of copper intra-uterine devices. *Int. J. Gynaecol. Obstet.* 14:341, 1976.

29. Kellogg, S. G.; Davis, C., and Benirschke, K. Candida parapsilosis: previously unknown cause of fetal infection. *J. Reprod. Med.* 12:159, 1974.

30. Last, P. A. Pregnancy and the intrauterine contraceptive device. *Contraception* 9:439, 1974.

31. Layde, P. M.; Goldberg, M. F.; Safra, M. J.; and Oakley, G. P. Failed intrauterine device contraception and limb reduction deformities: a case-control study. *Fertil. Steril.* 31:18, 1979.

32. Leighton, P. C.; Evans, D. G.; and Wallis, S. M. IUD and congenital malformation. *Br. Med. J.* 1:959, 1976.

33. Madrigal, V.; Thomas, M. N.; Goldsmith, A.; and Edelman, D. A. A two-year evaluation of the Dalkon Shield intrauterine device in San Salvador. Paper presented at the VII World Congress on Fertility and Sterility, Buenos Aires, Argentina, 3–9 November, 1974.

34. Matthews, J. Dalkon Shield: mid-trimester septic abortion. *Med. J. Australia* 2:856, 1974.

35. McCracken, J. S. IUD and congenital malformation. *JAMA* 1:1020, 1976.

36. Misenhimer, H. R., and Garcia-Bunuel, R. Failure of intrauterine contraceptive device and fungal infection in the fetus. *Obstet. Gynecol.* 34:368, 1969.

37. Monif, G. R. G.; D'Alessandri, R. M.; Khakoo, R. A.; and Kluge, R. M. Fatal sepsis associated with an intrauterine device and pregnancy. *South. Med. J.* 70: 249, 1977.

38. Mosley, W. H.; Chow, L. P.; and Liu, P. T. IUD related hospitalizations. A further analysis of device specific associations in the 1973 CDC study. Unpublished report from the Department of Population Dymanics, Johns Hopkins University, Baltimore, Maryland, 1974.

39. Neri, A.; Joel-Cohen, J.; and Ovadia, J. Ovarian abscess associated with incomplete abortion and intrauterine contraceptive device. *Isr. J. Med. Sci.* 13:305, 1977.

40. Propper, N. S., and Moore, J. H. Association of E. coli sepsis in pregnancy with a Cu-7 intrauterine device in place. *Obstet. Gynecol.* 48:76S, 1976 (Supplement).

41. Randic, L.; Ragab, I.; Thomas, M.; Kessel, E.; and Bernard, R. P. One-year evaluation of the spring coil IUD in Rijeka, Yugoslavia, and Cairo, Egypt. *Adv. Plann. Parent.* X:73, 1975.

42. Scott, R. B. Critical illnesses and deaths associated with intrauterine devices. *Obstet. Gynecol.* 31:322, 1968.

43. Sparks, R. A., and Letchworth, A. T. Mid-trimester septic abortion and *Escherichia coli* septicaemia in a copper IUCD user. *Br. Med. J.* 1:481, 1978.

44. Steven, J. D., and Fraser, I. S. The outcome of pregnancy after failure of an intrauterine contraceptive device. *J. Obstet. Gynaecol. Brit. Comnwlth.* 81: 282, 1974.

45. Stewart, W. C.; O'Brien, F. B.; Nissen, C.; and Deysach, L. Multiclinic evaluation of Gravigard (Cu 7) intrauterine contraception. In *Analysis of intrauterine contraception*, eds. F. Hefnawi and S. J. Segal. New York: American Elsevier Publishing Co., Inc., 1975.

46. Tatum, H. J.; Schmidt, F. H.; Phillips, D.; McCarty, M.; and O'Leary, W. M. The Dalkon Shield controversy: structural and bacteriological studies of IUD tails. *JAMA* 231:711, 1975.

47. Tatum, H. J.; Schmidt, F. H.; and Jain, A. K. Management and outcome of pregnancies associated with the Copper T intrauterine contraceptive device. *Am. J. Obstet. Gynecol.* 126:869, 1976.

48. Thomas, A. K. Septic abortion associated with a Lippes Loop. *Br. Med. J.* 3:747, 1975.

49. Tietze, C. Contraception with intrauterine devices 1959–1966. *Am. J. Obstet. Gynecol.* 96:1043, 1966.

50. Vessey, M.; Doll, R.; Peto, R.; Johnson, B.; and Wiggins, P. A long-term follow-up study of women using different methods of contraception—an interim report. *J. Biosoc. Sci.* 8:373, 1976.

51. Viechnicki, M. B. Septicemia and abortion with the Cu-7. *Am. J. Obstet. Gynecol.* 127:203, 1977.

52. Vujach, J., and Korman, B. Second trimester abortion and the Dalkon Shield. *Med. J. Australia* 2:249, 1975.

53. Wiles, C. M.; Cohens, S. L.; and Ward, R. H. T. Septic abortion and acute renal failure in a patient with an intra-uterine contraceptive device. *Int. J. Gynaecol. Obstet.* 15:464, 1978.

54. Wiles, P. J., and Zeiderman, A. M. Pregnancy complicated by intrauterine contraceptive devices. *Obstet. Gynecol.* 44:484, 1974.

55. Williams, P.; Johnson, B.; and Vessey, M. Septic abortion in women using intrauterine devices. *Br. Med. J.* 4:263, 1975.

56. Zuckerman, J. E., and Stubblefield, P. G. *E. coli* septicemia in pregnancy associated with the shield. *Am. J. Obstet. Gynecol.* 120:951, 1974.

Chapter 8
Ectopic pregnancy

Introduction

All women at risk of pregnancy are at risk of ectopic pregnancy. This risk includes those women who use a contraceptive method, such as an IUD, which does not always prevent conception. An undiagnosed, untreated ectopic pregnancy is a potentially life-threatening condition. Thirty-nine, or 10%, of the maternal deaths which occurred in the United States in 1976 were attributed to ectopic pregnancy (49).

In 1929, Gräfenberg (31) first mentioned that ectopic pregnancies may occur in women who use IUDs. The possibility that IUD users may be at a higher risk of ectopic pregnancy than nonusers did not become apparent until 1965, when Lippes (46) reported four ectopic pregnancies (17.4%) among 23 women who became pregnant with a Lippes Loop in situ. Since then, numerous published reports have discussed the possible association between IUD use and ectopic pregnancy, but none have provided the evidence necessary to determine whether or not IUDs cause ectopic pregnancies.

Incidence of Ectopic Pregnancy

Figure 8.1 shows the frequency of occurrence of ectopic pregnancies at different anatomical sites. Most

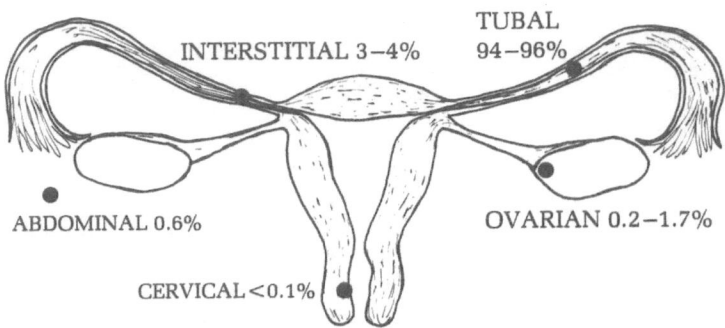

Figure 8.1: *The frequency of occurrence of ectopic pregnancies at different anatomical sites.*

ectopic pregnancies (94–96%) occur in the fallopian tube and an unknown number of these are aborted.

The ratios of ectopic pregnancies to deliveries and to total pregnancies as reported by various investigators are shown in Table 8.1. It is apparent that the usually quoted ratio of one ectopic pregnancy in every 200 pregnancies is probably a low estimate in the United States. The data presented in Table 8.1 vary substantially because most reports provide only the ratio of ectopic pregnancies to deliveries. Estimates of the ratio of ectopic pregnancies to total pregnancies have been based on the assumption that up to 20% of all pregnancies terminate in spontaneous abortion (18). The ratio of ectopic pregnancies to deliveries ranged from 1:28 to 1:264; the ratio of ectopic pregnancies to total pregnancies varied from 1:35 to 1:330. Whichever ratio is cited, the range of numbers reported suggests about a tenfold variation. The estimate of a 20% spontaneous abortion rate may be inaccurate, and therefore, the calculated ratios of ectopic to total pregnancies also may be inaccurate. In addition, the estimates of the ratio of ectopic pregnancies to total pregnancies do not reflect the numbers of women who have induced abortions. Unfortunately, data from abortion studies generally do not provide reliable estimates of the ratio of ectopic to intrauterine pregnancies.

Table 8.1 Ratios of ectopic pregnancy to deliveries and to total pregnancies.

Reference Number	Location/Year	Ectopic Pregnancy/ Deliveries	Ectopic Pregnancy/ Pregnancies
27	Baltimore, Maryland 1949–1953	1:215—whites (range 1:97–1:495) 1:166—blacks (range 1:34–1:905)	1:269 1:208
20	Indianapolis, Indiana 1936–1953	1:60	1:77
55	Lenoir, North Carolina 1950–1956	1:99	1:124
21	Jamaica, 1954–1961	1:28	1:35
9	New York, 1942–1957	1:64	1:80
11	Evanston, Illinois 1943–1962	1:233	1:253
75	New Orleans, Louisiana 1947–1963	1:116	1:145
13	New Jersey, 1947–1967	1:87	1:108
28	Atlanta, Georgia 1962–1970	1:118	1:148
47	Houston, Texas 1950–1952	1:264	1:330
36	California Oakland 1946–1951 Harbor 1957–1973 Fontana 1962–1973 Panorama 1962–1973 Beelflower 1962–1973 Los Angeles 1953–1972	1:105 1:155 1:260 1:212 1:161 1:100	1:143 1:195 1:326 1:266 1:202 1:125
29	Lackland, Texas 1965–1973	1:124	1:155
24	Turku, Finland 1966–1969 1970–1975	1:156 1:96	1:183 1:139

Among women undergoing therapeutic abortion, Seward and co-workers (63) reported an ectopic to intrauterine pregnancy ratio of 1:1591 among women not using an IUD. Schonberg (62) reported a ratio of 1:3796.

The ectopic to intrauterine pregnancy ratio in these studies probably is an accurate estimate of the true figure. The likelihood that a woman with an ectopic pregnancy would be included in a population of women who want abortions depends on the length of gestation at the time of abortion. Because women with ectopic pregnancies are usually treated early in gestation, these are removed from the population of women who may seek abortion later in pregnancy.

The data presented in Table 8.1 show sizeable variations in the incidence of ectopic pregnancy, most of which were reported before the widespread use of IUDs. If the factors responsible for these differences operate among IUD users as well as among the general population, then the variation in the incidence of ectopic pregnancy among IUD users also may be expected to show a wide variation. It may be reasonable to expect high ectopic pregnancy rates (determined as a percentage of pregnancies) among IUD users who become pregnant and who are living in an area where there is a high ectopic pregnancy rate among all women, and low IUD-associated ectopic pregnancy rates in areas where there is a low rate of ectopic pregnancy in the general population.

Several reports have suggested reasons for the apparent increase in the incidence of ectopic pregnancy during recent years.

Donovan (20), and more recently Schoen and Nowak (61), suggested that the increased incidence of ectopic pregnancy may be due to the more liberal use of antibiotics for the treatment of a variety of genital infections. Instead of the fallopian tubes becoming

completely closed as a result of infection, they remain patent but with impaired function as a result of
the late effects of inflammation and perhaps scarring.

Beral (6), in an epidemiologic study of the trends
in ectopic pregnancy in England and Wales, suggested that the increased use of IUDs might be a principal factor which has contributed to the increased
incidence of ectopic pregnancy observed in these
regions. Beral recognized that other factors might
also be contributory, namely the increase in the numbers of women having induced abortions or tubal
surgery or in those using progesterone-only oral contraceptives. The available data do not allow for an
adequate assessment of the contributions these sep-
arate factors may have made to the apparent increase
in the incidence of ectopic pregnancy because all of
these factors have been associated, at one time or
another, with an increased risk of ectopic pregnancy.

Erkkola and Liukko (24) attributed the increased
incidence of ectopic pregnancy in Turku, Finland, to
the increased use of IUDs in that area.

Demographic Risk Factors

The incidence of ectopic pregnancy is related to a
number of factors, including age, gravidity, history
of induced abortion, socioeconomic status and race.
Ectopic pregnancy is reported to occur more frequently among nonwhite women (27,68) and among
those of less affluent socioeconomic status (20); its
incidence is reported to increase with age and gravidity (68). Panayotou and co-workers (53) reported
a significantly higher relative risk of ectopic pregnancy among women with a history of prior induced
abortion than among those without induced abortions. At the present time, however, there is no
evidence to suggest that the association between
ectopic pregnancy and age, gravidity, race, socioeconomic status or prior induced abortion is any dif-

ferent for IUD users and for women who do not use
IUDs.

Other Risk Factors

It has been suggested that the following additional
factors may place women at an increased risk of ectopic pregnancy: PID, endometriosis, prior pelvic
surgery, abortion, retrograde menstruation, previous
ectopic pregnancy, uterine fibromas and structural
abnormalities of the fallopian tubes, such as diver-
ticulae.

Tubal reconstructive surgery, which is often
performed in an attempt to improve impaired fertility, increases the risk of subsequent ectopic pregnancy (64). With the possible exceptions of previous
ectopic pregnancy and prior PID, there has not been
an adequate assessment of the relative importance of
any specific factor or combination of factors as they
pertain to a predisposition to ectopic pregnancy. The
existence of one or more of these factors may, however, physiologically contribute to impaired tubal
function and thus to ectopic pregnancy.

> Persaud (56) compared the histologic appearance of
> fallopian tubes which were removed from women
> with ectopic pregnancies with those tubes removed
> from other women at the time of postpartum sterili-
> zation. Chronic inflammation and diverticulae with
> or without chronic inflammation were observed in a
> significantly higher proportion of tubes obtained at
> the time of surgery for ectopic pregnancies.

Infectious salpingitis is undoubtedly the single
most important risk factor for ectopic pregnancy.

> Bone and Greene (10) reviewed the literature in 1961
> and found that from 0.5% to 82.4% of the women
> with ectopic pregnancies reported a prior history of

salpingitis; at surgery, 8% to 50% of the women evidenced salpingitis based on gross examination and 19% to 95% evidenced salpingitis on microscopic examination of the excised tubes.

Westrom (77) provides further evidence in support of the widely held clinical impression that PID is an important factor in the etiology of ectopic pregnancy. Among 415 women who had laparoscopically confirmed diagnoses of PID and who were followed for 6 to 14 years, 263 had 449 pregnancies of which 19 were ectopic. This gave an ectopic to uterine pregnancy ratio of 1:24. The ratio was 1:147 for a control group of women with laparoscopic evidence of no PID at study admission.

Several recent studies have indicated that IUD users are at a greater risk of PID than women who do not use IUDs (see Chapter 4). It is not possible, however, to provide an adequate evaluation of the increased risk of ectopic pregnancy to IUD users with a history of PID without knowledge of the proportion of women with histories of PID who become pregnant with an IUD in situ and then have ectopic pregnancies.

Diagnosis and Management

The classic triad of symptoms for ectopic pregnancy is: amenorrhea, pain and tenderness. Unfortunately, these signs and symptoms are not specific for the diagnosis of ectopic pregnancy. Women with "delayed" menstrual periods, palpable pelvic masses, cervical tenderness on motion, pelvic or abdominal pain, rebound pain or tenderness and abnormal uterine bleeding all may lead to a tentative diagnosis of ectopic pregnancy. These signs and symptoms also are present with other conditions, so it is not surprising that ectopic pregnancy is often misdiagnosed as threatened or incomplete abortion, ovarian cysts (especially corpus luteum cysts), salpingitis and appendicitis.

Even if a patient's clinical history suggests pregnancy, a pregnancy test may not be helpful, especially if the gestation is very early. The production of human chorionic gonadotropin (HCG) is sometimes impaired in ectopic pregnancy and may be inadequate to support the endometrium. Many patients with ectopic pregnancies develop spotting or discharge as a result of irregular shedding of the endometrium. In these circumstances, uterine bleeding and/or a negative pregnancy test cannot necessarily rule out the possibility of early ectopic pregnancy. The recent introduction of more sensitive and specific assays for HCG, such as the radioimmunoassay or radioreceptor assay, enable an earlier and more accurate diagnosis of pregnancy than the standard immunologic slide or tube tests. However, even with the aid of a more sophisticated pregnancy test, the differential diagnosis between uterine and ectopic pregnancy is still necessary.

The diagnosis of ectopic pregnancy is further complicated in the IUD user because irregular bleeding episodes and pelvic and/or abdominal pain are known side effects of IUD use.

> Hallatt (36) has presented the difficulties involved in diagnosing ectopic pregnancy in IUD users. Ectopic pregnancy was not suspected in 70 women who had IUDs in situ and in whom ectopic pregnancy was eventually diagnosed. The symptoms of ectopic pregnancy were attributed to the IUD in 85% of the women: 28 of these women had their IUDs removed for pain and bleeding; another four had their IUDs removed and had others inserted.

Any delay in the diagnosis of ectopic pregnancy increases the likelihood of significant morbidity and mortality. Most deaths associated with ectopic pregnancy result from hemorrhage which occurs subsequent to rupture of the fallopian tube. Culdocentesis is often advocated when the diagnosis of ectopic pregnancy is suspected, because the presence of unclotted blood in the cul de sac is diagnostic of hemoperitoneum. Culdocentesis, however, is not necessarily diagnositc of ectopic pregnancy since hemoperitoneum can occur secondary to other causes, such as hemorrhagic corpus luteum, which may not require laparotomy for treatment. Whenever the physician strongly suspects an unruptured ectopic pregnancy, diagnostic laparoscopy is in order to confirm the diagnosis. If ruptured ectopic pregnancy is suspected, immediate laparotomy if indicated.

Ectopic Pregnancy Rates Among IUD Users

Ectopic pregnancy rates associated with various IUDs are usually reported as a percentage of pregnancies or, occasionally, as a Pearl Index. The drawback to using the percentage rate is that it does not take into account either the risk of becoming pregnant or the duration of follow-up. For example, a given IUD might be associated with a high pregnancy rate, but a small percentage of these pregnancies may be ectopic. In contrast, a second IUD may be associated with a low pregnancy rate, but a high percentage of these pregnancies may be ectopic. The actual risk of ectopic pregnancy, however, may be lower for the second IUD. Furthermore, as the duration of IUD use increases, the proportion of women with ectopic pregnancies may also be expected to increase.

Ectopic pregnancy rates calculated as a percentage of all pregnancies with the IUD in situ may lead some people to infer that the IUD causes ectopic pregnancy. Table 8.2 gives the expected percentage of ectopic pregnancies, assuming IUD failure rates of two and of four per 100 women per year, for different

Table 8.2 Relationship between ectopic pregnancy rates (EPR) in groups
of women not using contraceptives and of women using IUDs,

	No Contraceptives Used	IUDs used					
		No Decrease or Increase in EPR		Decrease of 25% in EPR		Increase of 25% in EPR	
	Expected number of pregnancies/100 women/year						
	80	2	4	2	4	2	4
EPR in General Population (%)	Expected number of ectopic pregnancies/ 100 women/year	Assumed change in EPR caused by IUD Expected percentage of pregnancies that will be ectopic					
		None		25%Decrease		25% Increase	
0.25 (1:400)	0.20	10.0	5.0	7.5	3.8	15.6	7.8
0.33 (1:300)	0.27	13.5	6.8	10.1	5.1	16.9	8.4
0.5 (1:200)	0.40	20.0	10.0	15.0	7.5	31.3	15.6
1.0 (1:100)	0.80	40.0	20.0	30.0	15.0	50.0	25.0
2.0 (1:50)	1.6	80.0	40.0	59.9	30.0	100.0	50.0

rates of ectopic pregnancy in the general population (0.25–2.0%). These percentages are based on the assumption that the IUD neither prevents nor causes ectopic pregnancy. Table 8.2 also shows that the expected percentage of pregnancies that are ectopic depends on the pregnancy rate of the IUD itself, as well as the pregnancy rate in the general population (assumed to be 80 per 100 women per year in a group of women not using contraceptives). The same calculations are repeated assuming the IUD 1) reduces the incidence of ectopic pregnancy by 25% and 2) increases the incidence of ectopic pregnancy by 25%.

The principal points illustrated in Table 8.2 are: 1) regardless of whether IUD users have the same, a higher or a lower ectopic pregnancy rate than a group of women not using contraceptives, the percentage of ectopic pregnancies in the group using IUDs will always be higher than that of the group not using contraceptives; 2) the higher percentage of pregnancies among IUD users does not imply that the IUD causes ectopic pregnancy.

The preferred method used to report ectopic pregnancy rates is the life table method (see Chapter 1). Unfortunately, none of the studies in the literature to date have used the life table method to report ectopic pregnancy rates. Ectopic pregnancy rates, expressed as Pearl indices, based on published reports are listed in Table 8.3. The data suggest that copper-bearing IUDs are associated with a lower rate of ectopic pregnancy and the progesterone-releasing IUDs with a higher rate of ectopic pregnancy than nonmedicated IUDs. The rates presented in Table 8.3 must be considered approximate, since the original reports do not always specify 1) the total woman-months of IUD use, 2) whether the diagnosis of ectopic pregnancy was confirmed by histologic exam-

Table 8.3 *Ectopic pregnancy rate for various IUDs.*

Reference Number		Woman-Years	Ectopic Pregnancies	Pearl Index (ectopic pregnancies/ 100 woman-years)
3	Progestasert	10,825	46	0.43
69	Lippes Loops Margulies Spiral Saf-T-Coil Birnberg Bow Steel Ring	28,614	34	0.12
74	Lippes Loops Saf-T-Coil M Dalkon Shield Cu-7 Others	9,768	10	0.10
25	Lippes Loop (All sizes)	6,895	9	0.13
67	Cu-7	21,800	9	0.04
51	Lippes Loop D	1,242	1	0.08
	Cu-7	1,242	1	0.08
	Cu-T-200	1,250	0	0.0
	Progestasert	960	2	0.21

Table 8.4 *Ectopic pregnancy rates (EPR) for different IUDs.*

IUD	Woman-Months of Use	EPR/100 Woman-Years
Cu-7	157,625	0.04
Cu-T	132,432	0.05
Nonmedicated	343,365	0.12
Progestasert	126,800	0.40

SOURCE: FDA drug bulletin (4)

ination or 3) whether the IUDs were in situ at the time pregnancy occurred. Moreover, differences in reported ectopic pregnancy rates may be related more closely to other risk factors, such as the prevalence of PID, which vary from population to population, than they are to the specific type of IUD.

In 1978, the United States Food and Drug Administration (FDA) convened a special meeting to assess the risks of ectopic pregnancy for different types of IUDs. Rates of ectopic pregnancy for different types of IUDs based on clinical data provided to the FDA are shown in Table 8.4. These rates are probably subject to the same limitations as those given in Table 8.3.

A rare form of ectopic pregnancy is ovarian pregnancy. Since the first such report by Piver and co-workers (57) in 1967, a total of 50 cases of ovarian pregnancy in association with an IUD in situ have been reported (5,8,11,15,16,19,22,23,26,30,32–34, 37,38,42–45,50,54,57–60,66,71–73) (Table 8.5). The data in Table 8.5 do not imply an increased risk of ovarian pregnancy for any specific type of IUD. The risk of ovarian pregnancy may be higher among IUD users compared to nonusers of IUDs who become pregnant. Lehfeldt and co-workers (44) reported that among IUD users 5 of 45 ectopic pregnancies were ovarian pregnancies. Gray and Ruffolo (33) found that for IUD users 4 of 8 ectopic pregnancies were ovarian pregnancies. The ratio of ovarian to ectopic pregnancies in the general population is estimated to be about 1:100.

Table 8.5 *Reports of ovarian pregnancy in association with IUD use.*

IUD	Ovarian Pregnancy Number of Cases
Lippes Loop	23
Dalkon Shield	4
Beospir	1
Cu-7	6
Cu-T	1
Birnberg Bow	1
Unspecified	14

Other rare forms of ectopic pregnancy include abdominal and cervical pregnancy.

Acker and co-workers (1), Clark and McMillan (17), Kasby and Krins (40), and Tisdall and co-workers (70) have reported five cases of abdominal pregnancy in patients with IUDs in situ; one IUD was a Lippes Loop, one a Cu-7, one a Saf-T-Coil, one a Dalkon Shield, and one in which the type of IUD was not specified.

We are unaware of any reports of cervical pregnancy with an IUD in situ.

Ectopic Pregnancy and Duration of IUD Use

Several investigators have reported that the ectopic pregnancy rate, determined as a percentage of pregnancies, increases as the duration of IUD use increases.

Vessey and co-workers (73) reported an increased rate of ectopic pregnancy after four years of IUD use: 2.6% for up to 24 months of IUD use compared to 27.3% for 49 or more months of IUD use.

Jain (41) reported a progressive increase in the ectopic pregnancy rates for Lippes Loop users which increased from 0.8% at one to 12 months to 4.0% for 37 or more months of IUD use.

Tatum and Schmidt (68) found that the percentage of ectopic pregnancies among Cu-T-200 users increased from 1.6% after 1 to 12 months of IUD use to 7.3% at 25 or more months of IUD use.

Tatum and Schmidt (68) postulated a causal relationship between the duration of IUD use and the occurrence of ectopic pregnancy. However, their analyses were based on ectopic pregnancy rates calculated as a percentage of pregnancies and not as a life-table rate; therefore, the inference of an increased risk of ectopic pregnancy with prolonged IUD use for any type of IUD is not necessarily correct.

If, as postulated by Lehfeldt and co-workers (44), the IUD offers the greatest contraceptive protection in the endometrial cavity, less in the fallopian tubes and none in the ovary, then it is reasonable to expect higher rates of ectopic pregnancy at sites distant from the uterus. This expectation has been confirmed in some reports but not in others.

Jonas (42) found that 24 of 75 (32.0%) ectopic pregnancies occurred in the interstitial and isthmic portion of the fallopian tubes in women who did not use IUDs and in none of the 11 ectopic pregnancies which occurred in individuals who had IUDs in situ.

Hallatt (36), on the other hand, reported almost identical rates of cornual, isthmic and ampullary implantations for 1,428 ectopic pregnancies in women who did not use IUDs and for 70 ectopic pregnancies among IUD users.

Ectopic Pregnancy and the IUD: Cause or Effect?

Since the publication of the report by Lippes (46) of a possible association between IUD use and ectopic pregnancy, numerous investigators have argued

about whether or not the IUD is a causative factor
in the etiology of ectopic pregnancy. It is apparent
from a review of the published data that women who
become pregnant with any type IUD in situ are at a
substantially higher risk of ectopic pregnancy than
women who do not use IUDs and who become pregnant. This fact does not necessarily implicate the
IUD in the etiology of ectopic pregnancy. If the IUD's
only antifertility mechanism is the prevention of the
blastocyst implantation, then it is reasonable to attempt to use a model in which the IUD is evaluated
in terms of the expected reduction of intrauterine
and ectopic pregnancies. An evaluation of this type
was made by Lehfeldt and co-workers (44) using
data reported by the Cooperative Statistical Program
(CSP) (69).

> Lehfeldt and co-workers (44) calculated that the
> IUD reduces the incidence of tubal pregnancy
> by 95%, but does not reduce the incidence of
> ovarian pregnancy. These estimates were based
> on approximately 45,000 woman-years of non-
> medicated IUD use as reported by the CSP in
> which there were 1,046 pregnancies with the
> IUD in situ, including 40 tubal and 5 ovarian
> pregnancies. The reduction in the incidence of
> tubal and ovarian pregnancy was calculated for
> a group of women not using contraceptives, as-
> suming a monthly fertilization rate of 30 per 100
> women per month, an ectopic pregnancy rate of
> 5 per 1,000 pregnancies and an ovarian preg-
> nancy rate of five per 1,000 ectopic pregnancies.
> The calculated reduction in tubal or ovarian
> pregnancies is dependent on these assumptions.
> There is some evidence that the ectopic preg-
> nancy rate may be considerably higher than
> 0.5% and the fertilization rate may be lower
> than 30 per 100 women per month, and there-
> fore, the reductions in tubal and ovarian preg-
> nancies which result from IUD use have been

Table 8.6 Expected reduction (%) in tubal and ovarian
          pregnancy rates due to IUD use, by ectopic pregnancy
          rate (EPR).

Type of Pregnancy by EPR (%)	Fertilization Rate/100 Women/Month	
	20	30
Tubal		
0.5	93.2	95.4
1.0	96.6	97.7
1.5	97.7	98.5
2.0	98.3	98.9
Ovarian		
0.5	NR*	NR*
1.0	14.5	43.0
1.5	43.0	62.0
2.0	57.3	71.5

*NR = no reduction

recalculated in Table 8.6. The expected reduction in tubal and ovarian pregnancies varies
considerably depending upon the assumed ectopic and fertilization rates. The data in Table
8.6 show that IUDs are more effective in pre-
venting tubal than ovarian pregnancy; they also
may prevent ovarian pregnancy, depending on
the assumptions made.

If the IUD indeed causes ectopic pregnancy,
then it would be reasonable to expect ectopic pregnancy rates to parallel uterine pregnancy rates for
the IUD, regardless of all other factors. In Table 8.7
intrauterine and ectopic pregnancy rates are shown
for the Progestasert based on international field
trials. While there is less than a two-fold difference
in the intrauterine pregnancy rates (1.3–2.3 per 100
woman-years), the ectopic pregnancy rates vary from
0.1 to 1.0 per 100 woman-years. This much greater
variation (10 times) of ectopic rates suggests that factors other than differences in IUDs must be taken
into account when comparing ectopic pregnancy
rates. Conception and ectopic pregnancy rates vary

from population to population. The data presented
in Table 8.7 afford some explanation as to why different ectopic pregnancy rates have been reported
for the same IUD when it is evaluated in different
populations.

The spectrum of the possible mechanisms of action of nonmedicated and medicated IUDs was reviewed in Chapter 1. It has not been absolutely
established that the IUD allows fertilization to occur,
but then prevents implantation. Some mechanisms
of action are common to a variety of IUDs (nonmedicated, copper-bearing, progesterone-releasing),
while others are specific for a given type of IUD. It
seems reasonable to assume that fertilization rates
may be different for specific types of IUDs. A higher
fertilization rate may be reflected in a higher ectopic
pregnancy rate in relation to the intrauterine pregnancy rate for a specific IUD. Once fertilization occurs, the fertilized ovum may implant outside the
uterus, in the uterus, or may reach the uterine cavity
but be unable to implant due to IUD-induced
changes in the uterine environment. The relative
frequency of each of these events may be different for
different IUDs. It is not possible to compute the
theoretical risk of ectopic pregnancy caused by a

Table 8.7 *Rates of uterine and ectopic pregnancy for the
Progestasert by geographic area.*

	Pearl Index (Pregnancies/ 100 Woman-Years)	
Geographic Area	Uterine Pregnancy	Ectopic Pregnancy
Eastern Canada	1.8	1.0
Scandinavia	2.3	0.9
California	1.6	0.6
Other Europe	2.1	0.6
Other United States	1.7	0.3
Latin America	1.3	0.1
Far East	1.4	0.0

SOURCE: Alza Corporation, unpublished data (3).

particular IUD without knowledge of these relative frequencies.

Iffy (40) has proposed the "menstrual reflux theory" as a possible cause of ectopic pregnancy. This theory hypothesizes that uterine bleeding, which occurs after fertilization but before implantation, acts either to impede the ovum's transport through the tube or displaces it from the uterus to an ectopic site. This theory also postulates that failure of the ovum to implant results from delayed ovulation followed by a shortened luteal phase of the menstrual cycle. Coincidentally, a shortened luteal phase of the menstrual cycle has been reported among some users of the Lippes Loop and the Cu-T-200 (14,48,52). It is not known whether the early onset of menstrual bleeding in IUD users places them at an increased risk of ectopic pregnancy as proposed by Iffy's menstrual reflux theory.

The interaction of IUDs with other risk factors for ectopic pregnancy also needs to be taken into account when exploring the possibility that the IUD may "cause" ectopic pregnancy. Chapter 4 reviews the association between IUD use and PID, and concludes that IUD users generally appear to be at a higher risk of PID than women who do not use IUDs, although it is not possible to associate any specific IUD with higher rates of PID than any other.

One limitation to any evaluation of the relationship between PID and ectopic pregnancy is that PID is sometimes asymptomatic, and a patient's recall of her medical history is not always accurate.

Weekes and Hutchins (76) found that 16.3% of 43 women with ectopic pregnancies gave a history of a previous pelvic infection, but 53.5% of the women had macroscopic or histologic evidence of a previous infection.

To our knowledge, no studies have been reported which compare ectopic pregnancy rates among

IUD users with a history of PID to those with no such history.

The Progestasert and Ectopic Pregnancy

Recently published data have implied that women who use the Progestasert have a higher risk of ectopic pregnancys than women who use copper-bearing or nonmedicated IUDs.

> Snowden (65) reported a 6- to 7-fold increased risk of ectopic pregnancy for women who used the Progestasert than for women who used copper-bearing IUDs or Lippes Loops when the ectopic pregnancy rate was determined either as a Pearl Index or as a percentage of pregnancies.
>
> Tatum and Schmidt (68) reviewed ectopic pregnancy rates and reported that 16.3% of the pregnancies which occurred with the Progestasert were ectopic. Ectopic pregnancies accounted for 5.1% of the pregnancies which occurred with an IUD of the same configuration which did not release progesterone, and for approximately 5% of the pregnancies which occurred with other IUDs.

Life table ectopic rates were not given in either of the above studies. Neither established a significantly higher risk of ectopic pregnancy for Progestasert users than for users of other types of IUDs.

In a double-blind, multi-center study of the Progestasert and the placebo Progestasert, only 1 of 45 pregnancies with the placebo Progestasert was ectopic compared to 1 of 8 pregnancies with the Progestasert (3). These rates, however, are not significantly different (p>0.10). In this study, the women were randomly assigned to one of the two IUDs and it can be assumed that the distribution of those factors which may place women at a higher risk of ectopic pregnancy were the same for both groups of study subjects. Further double-blind trials of the Progestasert and placebo Progestasert would be required to establish unequivocally the risk of ectopic pregnancy for these two IUDs. Such studies are probably not ethical in view of the unacceptably high failure rate associated with the placebo Progestasert (one year net life-table pregnancy rate 11.4 per 100 women). It is unlikely, therefore, that such studies will be conducted in the future.

Summary

Confusion over whether IUDs cause an increased risk of ectopic pregnancies stems from the findings that 2 to 5% of the pregnancies conceived with the nonmedicated or copper-bearing IUD in situ have been ectopic. In contrast, the rate of ectopic pregnancy in a noncontracepting group of women is usually stated to be 0.5%. These data have been used to infer that the IUD user is at a substantially higher risk of ectopic pregnancy than is the nonuser.

The data that have been presented in the literature to date are insufficient to demonstrate a causal relationship between IUD use and ectopic pregnancy. However, if the IUD user does become pregnant, she is at a higher risk of ectopic pregnancy than the woman who does not use an IUD.

References

1. Acker, O.; Jenson, A. B.; and Tenn, G. K. Abdominal pregnancy with intrauterine device *in situ. Obstet. Gynecol.* 42:36, 1973.

2. Ajjimakorn, S. Primary ovarian pregnancy IUD *in situ. J. Med. Assoc. Thai.* 58:1223, 1975.

3. Alza Corporation, Unpublished data. Palo Alto, California, 1978.

4. Anonymous. Progestasert IUD and ectopic pregnancy. FDA Drug Bulletin 8(6):37, 1979.

5. Basak, S.; Konar, M.; and Sinha, B. Ovarian pregnancy with Cu-T—A case report. Abstract in *Proceedings of First Asian Congress of Fertility and Sterility*, 19–23 February, Bombay, India, 1977.

6. Beral, V. An epidemiological study of recent trends in ectopic pregnancy. *Br. J. Obstet Gynaecol.* 82:775, 1975.

7. Berger, B. and Blechner, J. N. Ovarian pregnancy associated with Copper-7 intrauterine device. *Obstet. Gynecol.* 52:597, 1978.

8. Bjorn, G., and Jensen, H. K. Ovarian pregnancy. Report of a case with Lippes' Loop *in situ. Acta Obstet. Gynecol.* (Scand) 49:297, 1970.

9. Bobrow, M. L., and Bell, H. G. Ectopic pregnancy: a 16-year survey of 905 cases. *Obstet Gynecol.* 20:500, 1962.

10. Bone, N. L., and Greene, R. R. Histologic study of uterine tubes with tubal pregenancy. *Am. J. Obstet. Gynecol.* 82:1166, 1961.

11. Boronow, R. C.; McElin, T. W.; West, R. H.; and Buckingham, J. C. Ovarian pregnancy. Report of four cases and a thirteen-year survey of the English literature. *Am. J. Obstet. Gynecol.* 91:1095, 1965.

12. Bozza, A. T., and Horwitz, S. T. Ovarian pregnancy with an intrauterine contraceptive device *in situ:* a case report. *Am. J. Obstet. Gynecol.* 117:285, 1973.

13. Breen, J. L. A 21 survey of 654 ectopic pregnancies. *Am. J. Obstet. Gynecol.* 106:1004, 1970.

14. Brenner, P. F., and Mishell, D. R. Progesterone and estradiol patterns in women using an intrauterine contraceptive device. *Obstet. Gynecol.* 46:456, 1975.

15. Campbell, J. S.; Conklin, F. J.; Chang, V. Y. H.; Singh, K. C.; and Hurteau, G. D. Ovarian apoplexy, ovarian pregnancy and the IUCD. *Eur. J. Obstet. Gynecol. Reprod. Biol.* 3:3, 1973.

16. Campbell, J. S.; Hacquebard, S.; Mitton, D. M.; Hurteau, G. D.; Bobra, S. T.; and Sirois, J. Acute hemoperitoneum, IUD, and occult ovarian pregnancy. *Obstet. Gynecol.* 43:438, 1974.

17. Clark, A. D., and McMillan. Maternal death due to primary peritoneal pregnancy. *J. Obstet. Gynaecol. Brit. Comnwlth.* 81:652, 1974.

18. Danforth, D. N., ed. *Obstetrics gynecology.* 3rd ed. Hagerstown, Maryland: Harper & Row, Publishers, Inc., 1977.

19. Darwish, D. H., and Saafan, S. T. A. Ovarian ectopic pregnancy with IUCD. *Br. Med. J.* 4:143, 1975.

20. Donovan, W. H. Ectopic pregnancy in relation to maternal mortality. *Obstet. Gynecol.* 7:694, 1956.

21. Douglas, C. P. Tubal ectopic pregnancy. *Br. Med. J.* 2:838, 1963.

22. Dreishpoon, I. H. Complications of pregnancy with an intrauterine contraceptive device *in situ.* *Am. J. Obstet. Gynecol.* 121:412, 1975.

23. Duckman, S.; Suarez, J.; and Tantakesem, P. Ovarian pregnancy and the intrauterine contraceptive device. *Am. J. Obstet. Gynecol.* 118:570, 1974.

24. Erkkola, R., and Liukko, P. Intrauterine device and ectopic pregnancy. *Contraception* 16:569, 1977.

25. Family Planning Research Unit. *General assessment of the Lippes Loop intrauterine device.* Report no. 19. Exeter: University of Exeter, 1977.

26. Fernandez, C. M., and Barbosa, J. J. Primary ovarian

pregnancy and the intrauterine device. *Obstet. Gynecol.* 47:9S, 1976, Supplement.

27. Fontanilla, J., and Anderson, G. W. Further studies on the racial incidence and mortality of ectopic pregnancy. *Am. J. Obstet. Gynecol.* 70:312, 1955.

28. Franklin, E. W.; Zeiderman, A. M.; and Laemmle, P. Tubal ectopic pregnancy: etiology and obstetric and gynecologic sequelae. *Am. J. Obstet. Gynecol.* 117: 220, 1973.

29. Gilstrap, L. C., and Harris, R. E. Ectopic pregnancy: a review of 122 cases. *South. Med. J.* 69:604, 1976.

30. Girard, Y.; Behamdouni, M.; and LaRose, J-C. Primary ovarian pregnancy associated with the Dalkon Shield IUD. *Obstet. Gynecol.* 51:52S, 1978 (Suppl).

31. Gräfenberg, E. Die intrauterine method der konzeption-suerhutung. In *Intrauterine contraceptive rings: history and statistical appraisal.* III Congress World League for Sexual Reform. International Congress Series, no. 54. Amsterdam: Excerpta Medica, 1929.

32. Graff, G.; Lancet, M.; and Czernobilsky, B. Ovarian pregnancy with intrauterine devices *in situ.* *Obstet. Gynecol.* 40:535, 1972.

33. Gray, C. L., and Ruffolo, E. H. Ovarian pregnancy associated with intrauterine contraceptive devices. *Am. J. Obstet. Gynecol.* 132:134, 1978.

34. Green, S., and Hinkle, D. Experiences with IUD complications. *Tex. Med.* 66:60, 1970.

35. Hallatt, J. G. Repeat ectopic pregnancy: a study of 123 consecutive cases. *Am. J. Obstet. Gynecol.* 122:520, 1975.

36. Hallatt, J. G. Ectopic pregnancy associated with the intrauterine device: a study of seventy cases. *Am. J. Obstet. Gynecol.* 125:754, 1976.

37. Harris, W. H. Ovarian pregnancy associated with an intrauterine device. *Can. Med. Assoc. J.* 104:531, 1971.

38. Helde, M. D.; Campbell, J. S.; Himaya, A.; Nuyens, A. J. J.; Cowley, F. C.; and Hurteau, G. D. Detection of unsuspected ovarian pregnancy by wedge resection. *Can. Med. Assoc. J.* 107:237, 1972.

39. Horne, H. W., and Scott, J. M. Intrauterine contraceptive devices in women with proven fertility: a 5-year follow-up study. *Fertil. Steril.* 20:400, 1969.

40. Iffy, L. The role of premenstrual, post-mid-cycle conception in the aetiology of ectopic pregnancy. An evaluation of the reflux theory. *J. Obstet. Gynaecol. Br. Comnwlth.* 70:996, 1963.

41. Jain, A. K. Non-medicated intrauterine devices: review and assessment. Paper presented at a WHO Symposium on Advances in Fertility Regulation, 16—19 November, 1976, Moscow, USSR.

42. Jonas, G. Ectopic pregnancy despite intrauterine contraception: a clue to mode of action of I.U.C.D.s. *Br. Med. J.* 2:467, 1975.

43. Kasby, C., and Krins, A. Primary peritoneal pregnancy in association with intrauterine contraceptive devices: two case reports. *Brit. J. Obstet. Gynaecol.* 85:794, 1978.

44. Lehfeldt, H.; Tietze, C.; and Gorstein, F. Ovarian pregnancy and the intrauterine device. *Am. J. Obstet. Gynecol.* 108:1005, 1970.

45. Levin, S.; Caspi, E.; and Hirsch, H. Ovarian pregnancy and intrauterine devices. *Am. J. Obstet. Gynecol.* 113:843, 1972.

46. Lippes, J. Contraception with intrauterine plastic loops. *Am. J. Obstet. Gynecol.* 93:1024, 1965.

47. Lucci, J. A. Ectopic pregnancy. An analysis of 70 cases. *Am. J. Obstet. Gynecol.* 66:1178, 1953.

48. Martin, P. M.; and Brown, J. B. The effect of intra-
    uterine contraceptive devices on ovarian and men-
    strual function in the human. *J. Clin. Endocrinol.
    Metab.* 36:1125, 1973.

49. National Center for Health Statistics. *Monthly vital sta-
    tistics report. Final monthly statistics,* 1976. vol. 26,
    no. 2, Supplement (2), March 30, 1978.

50. Neuenschwander, M. F. Ovarialgraviditat bei intra-
    uterinpessar. *Schweiz Ges Gynak. Jahresvers.* Crans,
    Switzerland, 1971.

51. Newton, J. R., Ectopic pregnancy and IUDs. *Br. J. Fam.
    Plann.* 3:78, 1978.

52. Nygren, K-G., and Johansson, E. D. B. Premature on-
    set of menstrual bleeding during ovulatory cycles in
    women with an intrauterine contraceptive device.
    Am. J. Obstet. Gynecol. 117:971, 1973.

53. Panayotou, P. P.; Kaskarelis, D. B.; Miettinen, O. S.;
    Trichopoulos, D. B.; and Kalandidi, A. K. Induced
    abortion and ectopic pregnancy. *Am. J. Obstet. Gyne-
    col.* 114:507, 1972.

54. Pane, A.; Sabatalle, R.; and Rayniak, J. V. Ovarian preg-
    nancy with *in situ* IUCD: report of two cases. *Am. J.
    Obstet. Gynecol.* 108:672, 1970.

55. Parker, S. L., and Parker, R. T. "Chronic" ectopic preg-
    nancy. *Am. J. Obstet. Gynecol.* 74:1174, 1957.

56. Persaud, V. Etiology of tubal ectopic pregnancy.
    Radiologic and pathologic studies. *Obstet. Gynecol.*
    36:257, 1970.

57. Piver, M. S.; Baer, K. A.; and Zachary, T. V. Ovarian
    pregnancy and intrauterine device. *JAMA* 201:323, 1967.

58. Pugh, W. E.; Vogt, R. F.; and Gibson, R. A. Primary
    ovarian pregnancy and the intrauterine device. *Obstet.
    Gynecol.* 42:218, 1973.

59. Rimdusit, P., and Kasatri, N. Primary ovarian pregnancy and the intrauterine contraceptive device. *Obstet. Gynecol.* 48:575, 1976 (Supplement).

60. Robertson, S. Ovarian pregnancy in association with a "Copper 7" intrauterine device. *Aust. N.Z. J. Obstet. Gynaecol.* 14:48, 1974.

61. Schoen, J. A., and Nowak, R. J. Repeat ectopic pregnancy. A 116-year clinical survey. *Obstet. Gynecol.* 45:542, 1975.

62. Schonberg, L. A. Ectopic pregnancy and first trimester abortion. *Obstet. Gynecol.* 49:73S, 1977 (Supplement).

63. Seward, P. N.; Israel, R.; and Ballard, C. A. Ectopic pregnancy and intrauterine contraception: a definite relationship. *Obstet. Gynecol.* 40:214, 1972.

64. Siegler, A. M. Surgical treatment for tuboperitoneal causes of infertility since 1967. *Fertil. Steril.* 28:1019, 1977.

65. Snowden, R. The Progestasert and ectopic pregnancy. *Br. Med. J.* 2:1600, 1977.

66. Stahmann, F. S. Primary ovarian pregnancy with IUD. *S.D. J. Med.* 92:23, 1969.

67. Stewart, W. C.; O'Brien, F. B.; Nissen, C.; and Deysach, L. Multiclinic evaluation of Gravigard (Cu 7) intrauterine contraception. In *Analysis of intrauterine contraception,* eds. F. Hefnawi and S. J. Segal. New York: American Elsevier Publishing Co., Inc., 1975.

68. Tatum, H. J., and Schmidt, F. H. Contraceptive and sterilization practices and extrauterine pregnancy: a realistic perspective. *Fertil. Steril.* 28:407, 1977.

69. Tietze, C., and Lewit, S. Evaluation of intrauterine devices: ninth progress report of the Cooperative Statistical Program. *Stud. Fam. Plann.* July, 1970.

70. Tisdall, L. H.; Nichols, R. A.; and Sicuranza, B. J. Abdominal pregnancy associated with an intrauterine device. *Am. J. Obstet. Gynecol.* 106:937, 1970.

71. Varga, L.; Metz, I.; and Steiger, E. Another case of ovarian pregnancy in a patient with IUD. *Arch. Fur. Gynaecol.* 217:289, 1974.

72. Varga, L.; Obolensky, W.; and Scheidegger, S. Ovarian pregnancy and the intra-uterine device (IUD). A case report. *Int. J. Fertil.* 17:142, 1972.

73. Vessey, M. P.; Doll, R.; Johnson, B.; and Peto, R. Outcome of pregnancy in women using an intrauterine device. *Lancet* I:495, 1974.

74. Vessey, M.; Doll, R.; Peto, R.; Johnson, B.; and Wiggins, P. A long-term follow-up study of women using different methods of contraception—an interim report. *J. Biosoc. Sci.* 8:373, 1976.

75. Webster, H. D.; Barclay, D. L.; and Fischer, C. K. Ectopic pregnancy. A seventeen-year review. *Am. J. Obstet. Gynecol.* 92:23, 1965.

76. Weekes, A. R. L., and Hutchins, C. J. Ectopic pregnancy: a five year review. *Br. J. Clin. Pract.* 30:104, 1976.

77. Westrom, L. Effect of acute pelvic inflammatory disease on fertility. *Am. J. Obstet. Gynecol.* 121:707, 1975.

Chapter 9

Return to fertility after IUD discontinuation

Introduction

Most women use IUDs to space their pregnancies
rather than as a permanent means of fertility control.
The IUD is expected to be a temporary and reversible
contraceptive method which will have no long-term
adverse effects on subsequent reproductive function.
An immediate return to fertility is anticipated following removal of the device.

Return to Fertility

Most women who have their IUDs removed because
they wish to become pregnant usually experience
a rapid return to fertility, regardless of the type of
IUD used.

Sakurabayashi (7) reported that 80.0% of 35 women
conceived within 14 months after the removal of
polyethelene ring IUDs.

Wajntraub (12) followed 305 women who had
intrauterine rings removed in order to conceive;
74.1% conceived within six months and 86.8% within 12 months of IUD removal. Conception rates were
similar for women aged 18 to 30 and for women aged
31 to 44. Consistently lower conception rates were
obtained for women who had used intrauterine rings
for 19 to 36 months (80.0% after 12 months) than for

223

women who had used them for 1 to 18 months (85.8% after 12 months).

Tietze (9) studied 611 women who had their IUDs (Lippes Loop, Margulies Spiral, Birnberg Bow, steel ring, Saf-T-Coil) removed for planned pregnancies and found that 77.0% conceived within six months and 88.3% within 12 months of IUD removal. Conception rates were similar for women aged 17 to 25 and for women aged 26 to 42, as well as for women who had used their IUDs for less than 20 months or for 20 or more months.

The cumulative conception rates for 554 women who had Cu-T IUDs removed to become pregnant were not significantly different for women who had used the IUD for less than or more than one year (6). The cumulative conception rates after IUD removal (life table) were 77 per 100 women at six months and 92 per 100 women at 12 months.

Of 154 women who had their Progestasert IUDs removed to become pregnant, the cumulative conception rate (life table) at 12 months was 76 per 100 women (1).

Kaye and co-workers (5) followed 36 women after removal of Lippes Loops, Saf-T-Coils, Dalkon Shields or Cu-7s. Twelve months after removal, 88.9% had conceived. Conception rates appeared to be independent of the type of IUD used and duration of use.

The rates of conception for women who have their IUDs removed to become pregnant do not appear to depend either on the duration of IUD use or on the type of IUD. One limitation to these reports, however, is that they restrict attention to the subsequent fertility of a select group of IUD users and do not include the large numbers of women who discontinue IUD use for medical reasons, which includes women with either frank or subclinical PID. To our knowledge, there are no studies which have evaluated the subsequent fertility of these women. It remains to be established whether their fertility following IUD removal is the same as it is following elective removal for planned pregnancy.

The 12-month conception rate of women who discontinue IUD use to become pregnant appears to be higher than the rate for women who discontinue oral or injectable contraceptives, and similar to the rate of women who discontinue barrier contraceptives.

> Ellinas (3) reported the following 12-month conception rates for women discontinuing various types of contraception: IUD (types not specified), 96.8%; diaphragm, 91.2%; oral contraceptives, 87.0%; Depo-Provera (medroxyprogesterone acetate), 82.8%.

> The prospective study of the British Family Planning Association evaluated the proportion of parous women who delivered a live birth or stillbirth within 12 months of terminating various contraceptive methods. The results were as follows: oral contraceptives, 40.1%; diaphragm, 64.8%; IUD, 51.5%; and other methods of contraception, 61.8%. However, by 24 months after contraceptive discontinuation, the percentages of women remaining undelivered were similar for all methods of contraception (10).

Outcome of Pregnancy After IUD Discontinuation

There is no evidence to indicate that the outcomes of planned pregnancies conceived after the elective removal of IUDs are different from the outcome of pregnancies which follow the discontinuation of other contraceptive methods.

> Vessey and co-workers (10) found similar birth weights and rates of live birth (normal and malformed), stillbirth, spontaneous abortion and ectopic

pregnancy among 1,281 planned pregnancies of previously parous women who had not practiced contraception or who had discontinued various contraceptive methods or practices (orals, diaphragm, IUD—principally Lippes Loops and Saf-T-Coils).

It has been suggested, but not confirmed, that there is a possibility of an increased risk of ectopic pregnancy after the discontinuation of IUD use. Tatum and Schmidt (8) reported seven (1.0%) ectopic pregnancies among 671 planned pregnancies following the removal of Cu-Ts. Vessey and co-workers (10) reported no ectopic pregnancies among 121 women who conceived after IUD discontinuation.

The ectopic pregnancy rate following IUD discontinuance becomes meaningful only when it is compared to the ectopic pregnancy rate of the general population where each IUD study is conducted. The rate may be influenced, for example, by the prevalence of PID in a specific population. The ectopic pregnancy rate reported by Tatum and Schmidt (8) is not excessive when compared to the ectopic pregnancy rate in the general population (see Chapter 8, Table 8.1).

Pelvic Infection and Infertility

The leading cause of involuntary infertility among women in the United States is tubal disease subsequent to pelvic infection. There is no reason to expect that women who acquire PID while using an IUD are any more or less likely to experience subsequent infertility than are women who do not use IUDs.

Westrom (13) evaluated pregnancy rates in 415 women who had laparoscopically confirmed diagnoses of acute salpingitis and in 100 control subjects who underwent laparoscopy, but did not have salpingitis. None of the women had any abnormalities which were known to impair fertility. All women were followed for 6 to 14 years (mean, 9.5 years). The overall infertility rate was 21.5% when the voluntarily childless and those who were involuntarily childless for reasons other than tubal occlusion were excluded. The infertility rates attributable to tubal occlusion among women who had 1, 2, 3 or more prior tubal infections were 12.9, 35.5, and 75.0%, respectively. The rate in the control group was 3.4%. Among women who had a single instance of acute gonorrheal infection, 6.1% were involuntarily childless compared to 17.3% of those with nongonococcal PID.

The studies reviewed in Chapter 4 indicated that women who use IUDs are at a higher risk of pelvic infection than women who do not. Therefore, the IUD user also may be at an increased risk of subsequent infertility as a result of damaged or occluded fallopian tubes.

Elstein (4) used hysterosalpingography to evaluate the incidence of damaged or occluded fallopian tubes in 50 IUD users subsequent to treatment of a pelvic infection. All women had been pregnant prior to IUD use. Evidence of bilateral tubal patency, as determined by free spillage of dye from both tubes, was demonstrated in only 12 (24.0%) women. Unilateral tubal occlusion was present in 16 (32.0%) women and bilateral tubal occlusion in seven (14.0%). Other evidence of tubal damage, such as delayed or localized spill and kinking or dilation of the tubes was evident in 15 (30.0%) women. In a control group (10 asymptomatic IUD users; eight Lippes Loops and two Saf-T-Coils), free bilateral spill was demonstrated in nine (90.0%) women.

Achari and Kundra (2) performed hysterosalpingographic evaluations of 100 parous women who had used an IUD for six months to three years. Bi-

lateral tubal blockage was present in 10% and unilateral tubal blockage in 5% of the women. The
proportion of women with bilateral tubal patency appeared to decrease as the duration of IUD use increased.

The results of the cited studies indicate high
rates of unilateral or bilateral tubal blockage after a
pelvic infection among IUD users, but they do not
establish whether these rates are higher than those
which occur among nonusers who acquire a pelvic
infection. Hysterosalpingographic studies do not
demonstrate all aspects of tubal function, either impaired or normal. The only unequivocal proof of in-
tact tubal function is intrauterine pregnancy.

Studies which have evaluated conception rates
subsequent to IUD discontinuation are inadequate to
establish rates of infertility which are specifically
caused by pelvic infections. For example, if it is assumed that 5 to 10% of all IUD users have pelvic
infections and that 20% of these women are infertile
as a result of the infection, then only 1 to 2% of the
women who discontinue IUD use in order to conceive will fail to conceive as a result of IUD-
associated PID. This small percentage of infertile
women will have a negligible effect on the overall
conception rate.

Summary

No published evidence suggests that IUDs impair
subsequent fertility to a greater degree than other
temporary methods of contraception. Studies which
have evaluated conception rates after elective IUD
removal indicate that their rates usually are independent of the type of IUD and the duration of use.
However, conception rates following IUD removal
for medical reasons, including PID, have not been

evaluated. The available evidence indicates that the outcome of pregnancies conceived after IUD removal are no different than the outcome of those which follow the cessation of most other contraceptive methods.

References

1. Alza Corporation. *The Progestasert*. Intrauterine progesterone contraceptive system release rated 65μg/day progesterone for one year. Alza Product Information, Palo Alto, California, 1977.

2. Achari, K., and Kundra, V. L. Hysterosalpingographic changes due to long term effect of intrauterine device. *J. Obstet. Gynaecol.* (India) XXIV:292, 1974.

3. Ellinas, S. P. Experience with medroxyprogesterone acetate (Depo-Provera) as an injectable contraceptive. *Int. J. Gynaecol. Obstet.* 15:145, 1977.

4. Elstein, M. The effects of pelvic inflammation associated with the IUD. *Int. J. Fertil.* 14:275, 1969.

5. Kaye, B. M.; Reaney, B. V.; Kaye, D. L.; and Edelman, D. A. Long-term safety and use-effectiveness of intrauterine devices. *Fertil. Steril.* 28:937, 1977.

6. Population Council. *Copper T Model TCu 200: summary of investigations*. New York: The Population Council, 1975.

7. Sakurabayashi, M. Experience with polyethylene ring: 1955–1965, part 1. *Yokohama Med. Bull.* 17:91, 1966.

8. Tatum, H. J., and Schmidt, F. H. Contraceptive and sterilization practices and extrauterine pregnancy: a realistic perspective. *Fertil. Steril.* 28:407, 1977.

9. Tietze, C. Fertility after discontinuation of intrauterine and oral contraception. *Int. J. Fertil.* 13:385, 1968.

10. Vessey, M.; Doll, R.; Peto, R.; Johnson, B.; and Wiggins, P. A long term follow-up study of women using different methods of contraception—an interim report. *J. Biosoc. Sci.* 8:373, 1976.

11. Vessey, M. P.; Wright, N. H.; McPherson, K.; and Wiggins, P. Fertility after stopping different methods of contraception. *Br. Med. J.* 1:265, 1978.

12. Wajntraub, G. Fertility after removal of the intrauterine ring. *Fertil. Steril.* 21:555, 1970.

13. Westrom, L. Effect of acute pelvic inflammatory disease on fertility. *Am. J. Obstet. Gynecol.* 121:707, 1975.

Chapter 10

IUD complications
in perspective

The last twenty years of research have resulted in major advancements and dramatic improvements in the field of intrauterine contraception. Thousands of papers and at least three books have focused on the safety and efficacy of IUDs. Intrauterine contraception has been the topic of countless presentations made at innumerable national and international conferences and workshops. In spite of this impressive quantity of work, basic questions of academic, research and clinical importance have not been answered adequately. The inadequacy of our present knowledge was underscored in 1977 when the United States Food and Drug Administration (FDA) held a special meeting to assess the risks of PID to IUD users. One year later, another special FDA meeting was held to evaluate the risks of ectopic pregnancy for users of various types of IUDs.

One of the pioneers in IUD development and research, Dr. Jaime Zipper, recently noted that a better understanding of the mechanism of action of IUDs was needed before further design developments could proceed in a rational manner (12). Although research on IUDs has continued extensively in recent years, the precise mechanisms through which IUDs exert their antifertility effects in the human are only partially known (see Chapter 1). For any type of IUD, the following three biological events are probably responsible for its antifertility effects: 1) interference with fertilization, 2) interference with blastocyst implantation and 3) early destruction (abortion) of the implanted blastocyst. Further research is required to determine the manner in which the IUD affects each of these biological events. The significance of IUD-induced changes in endometrial prostaglandin E and F levels, endometrial fibrinolytic activity, plasma immunoglobulin A, G and M levels, and the levels of uterine enzymes need to be further evaluated to determine the role, if any, of these changes in the antifertility effects and side effects of IUDs.

In addition to obtaining a clearer understanding of the antifertility effects of IUDs, future research should focus on the interrelationships between IUD use and the events which frequently lead to discontinuation, including expulsion and removal for pain and/or bleeding. When these relationships are delineated, it may be possible to base modifications of IUD design on a more solid foundation of facts than has been possible with the trial and error experimentation of the past.

The development and testing of new IUDs is being undertaken along the following lines:

1. Preliminary trials of IUDs with biodegradable extensions for use in the immediate postpartum period have indicated that such extensions added to either a Lippes Loop or Cu-T are effective in reducing the high expulsion rate associated with immediate postpartum insertions (2).
2. Preliminary results of research on synthetic hormone-releasing devices suggest that a d-norgestrel-releasing IUD (6,7,9) and a norethisterone-releasing IUD (8) may further reduce failure rates and undesired heavy uterine bleeding.
3. Research on IUDs which release microgram amounts of antifibrinolytic agents (10) suggests that these IUDs have diminished incidence rates of unpredictable uterine bleeding.

4. The use of heavy metals other than copper in IUDs is being explored. Medel and associates have shown that the addition of zinc to the Cu-T reduces the pregnancy rate when compared to the Cu-T alone (4).

Other approaches can be taken to improve IUD performance and acceptability. IUD performance may be improved by selectively fitting IUDs to individual patients (see Chapter 2). There is clearly a need to reduce IUD-related morbidity through the development of procedures which will identify women who are high-risk subjects and not suitable for an IUD insertion. While a number of medical contraindications are recognized for an IUD insertion (see Chapter 1), other factors may also preclude some women from using this form of contraception. Since most IUDs cause an increase in the amount of menstrual blood loss along with occasional spotting, consideration should be given to a woman's perceptions of her menstrual cycle and her acceptance of potential changes in her menstrual pattern. Similarly, given that IUD users are at a higher risk of PID than are nonusers, women with other known risk factors for PID, such as a prior history of the disease or multiple sex partners, should be carefully advised of their high-risk category and of the strong contraindications to their use of IUDs.

IUD morbidity may be minimized and performance maximized if careful attention is paid to the insertion procedure. Adequate training in the techniques of IUD insertion is essential. These techniques vary with the type of IUD, but an important principle of all IUD insertions is the correct fundal placement of the device within the uterine cavity.

The recognition of IUD-related complications and their prompt treatment can reduce serious morbidity or may prevent a potential mortality. This has been well illustrated in terms of IUD related abortion deaths.

Table 10.1 Theoretical (method) and actual (use) effectiveness rates of
different contraceptive methods.

	Correct and Consistent Use	Average US Experience Among 100 Women Who Wanted No More Children
	Theoretical (Method) Effectiveness	Actual (Use) Effectiveness
Abortion	0	0+
Tubal Ligation	0.04	0.04
Vasectomy	0.15	0.15+
Oral Contraceptives (combined)	0.34	4–10
Intramuscular Long-Acting Progestin	0.25	5–10
Low Dose Oral Progestin	1.0–1.5	5–10
IUD	1.0–3.0	5
Condom	3.0	10
Diaphragm with Spermicide	3.0	17
Spermicidal Foam	3.0	22
Coitus Interruptus	9.0	20–25
Rhythm (calendar)	13.0	21

NOTE: Table gives percentages of women who would become pregnant within one
year of initiation of the contraceptive method.
SOURCE: Hatcher, R. A., et al. (1).

Seventeen deaths were reported in the United
States from 1972 to 1974 for women who became
pregnant with an IUD in situ (see Chapters 4 and 7).
The association between IUD-related abortion deaths
was widely publicized in the mass media; since the
second half of 1974, only two deaths from IUD-associated spontaneous abortions have been reported. This
change has not been due solely to the withdrawal
of the Dalkon Shield from the market in June 1974.
Reported deaths associated with other IUDs, which
are still in use, have also practically disappeared.

None of the currently available methods of contraception is free of side effects, complications or
failure. The failure rates associated with IUDs are
low compared with those of other temporary methods
of fertility control (Table 10.1). Any consideration of
the overall safety of different contraceptive methods

must include an evaluation of what may happen to those women who become pregnant while using the method. Some pregnancies will spontaneously abort. Some women will elect to have their pregnancies terminated with an induced abortion, and others will carry their pregnancies to term. Regardless of the specific outcome of such pregnancies, all are associated with potential complications. For the most part, each contraceptive method is associated with a unique set of complications. It is therefore difficult to compare complication rates of different contraceptive methods. Tietze (11) has suggested that death is the only useful common denominator for the comparative evaluation of the risks to health of different contraceptive methods. Table 10.2 gives the combined risk of death for women in different age groups from causes due to specific contraceptive methods or to pregnancies which resulted from contraceptive method failures. This table shows that the risk of death associated with IUD use (particularly at older ages) is actually lower than it is for all other contraceptive methods when the mortality risk associated with unwanted pregnancy is taken into account.

One indirect measure of side effects and complications for different contraceptive methods is the continuation rate for each method. Continuation rates for IUD users in some studies have been shown to be higher than they are for oral contraceptive users.

Table 10.2 Death rates per 100,000 women attributable to different contraceptive methods.

Contraceptive Method	Age (Years)					
	15–19	20–24	25–29	30–34	35–39	40–44
None	5.6	6.1	7.4	13.9	20.8	22.6
Orals						
Nonsmokers	1.3	1.4	1.4	2.2	4.5	7.1
Smokers	1.5	1.6	1.6	10.8	13.4	58.9
IUDs	0.9	1.0	1.2	1.4	2.0	1.9
Barrier Methods	1.1	1.6	2.0	3.6	5.0	4.2

SOURCE: Tietze, C. (11).

Lippes and Feldman (3) compared the continuation rates of Lippes Loop users and oral contraceptive users. After one year of use, the continuation rates were similar for both groups. Continuation rates after two, three, four and five years, however, were higher for the Lippes Loop users (58.8 versus 38.0 per 100 women at five years). A similar finding was reported by Melton and Shelton (5). The one-year continuation rates for Dalkon Shield and oral contraceptive users were 69.9 and 55.4 per 100 women, respectively.

Obviously, differences among continuation rates by different methods of contraception are due to factors other than discontinuation for method-related reasons. Women discontinue contraceptive methods for various reasons that are often unrelated to the occurrence of adverse reactions associated with the method. It must also be recognized that a woman may independently discontinue the use of oral contraceptives at any time, but she must have the participation of the physician to remove an IUD.

Unfortunately, the ideal method of contraception does not presently exist. All methods have side effects, complications and failures. The IUD is one of several effective methods of contraception. It plays an important role in the armamentarium of contraceptive methods available to clinicians and patients. This volume has been devoted to an examination of various complications associated with IUD use. This in no way implies that the IUD is neither safe nor effective relative to other presently available contraceptive methods. Current knowledge, however, clearly indicates that the use of IUDs can be made safer by adherence to the following precautions.

1. Women must be screened carefully for any contraindication to IUD insertion and use.
2. The person who inserts the device must follow the correct insertion technique.

3. Women must be encouraged to report immediately any adverse effects to their physicians so that the IUD can be removed if necessary, and prompt treatment can be initiated.
4. Clinicians must be continually vigilant regarding the possible complications of all contraceptive methods. Any time a woman is seen in an emergency room, clinic or physician's office, she should be questioned about her method of contraception. Frequently, the diagnosis of a contraceptive-related complication is missed simply because the physician was unaware of the patient's contraceptive method.

References

1. Hatcher, R. A.; Stewart, G. K.; Stewart, F.; Guest, F.; Stratton, P.; and Wright, A. H. *Contraceptive technology 1978–1979, 9th revised ed.* New York: Irvington Publishers, Inc., 1978.

2. International Fertility Research Program, Unpublished data. Research Triangle Park, North Carolina.

3. Lippes, J., and Feldman, J. G. A five-year comparison of the continuation rates between women using Loop D and oral contraceptives. *Contraception* 3:313, 1971.

4. Medel, M.; Zipper, J.; Dabancens, A.; and Thomas, M. Contraceptive efficacy of two different metals using a modified seven vector. *Int. J. Gynaecol. Obstet.* 14: 494, 1976.

5. Melton, R. J., and Shelton, J. D. Pill versus IUD: continuation rates of oral contraceptive and Dalkon Shield users in Maryland clinics. *Contraception* 4:319, 1971.

6. Nilsson, C. G.; Johansson, E. D. B.; and Luukkainen, T. A d-Norgestrel-releasing IUD. *Contraception* 13:503, 1976.

7. Nilsson, C. G. Comparative quantification of menstrual blood loss with a d-Norgestrel-releasing IUD and a nova-T-copper device. *Contraception* 15:379, 1977.

8. Nilsson, C. G.; Luukkainen, T.; and Lahteenmaki, P. Contraception with a Norethisterone-releasing IUD. Plasma levels of Norethisterone and its influence on the ovarian function. *Contraception* 17:115, 1978.

9. Nilsson, C. G.; Luukkainen, T.; and Lahteenmaki, P. Determination of plasma concentrations of d-Norgestrel during a one year follow-up in women with a d-Norgestrel-releasing IUD. *Contraception* 17:569, 1978.

10. Ragab, M. I., and Thomas, M. N. The use of tranexamic acid (AMCA) in IUDs as an anti-bleeding agent. *Int. J. Gynaecol. Obstet.* 14:137, 1976.

11. Tietze, C. What price fertility control? Lower than that of unwanted pregnancy. *Contemp. Obstet. Gynecol.* 12(1):32, 1978.

12. Zipper, J.; Edelman, D. A.; and Goldsmith, A. An overview of IUD research and implications for the future. *Int. J. Gynaecol. Obstet.* 15:73, 1977.

Appendix A

The studies listed in this appendix are a selected sample of studies which have reported on uterine perforations in association with IUD use. The studies were selected to give the reader an indication of the variability of the reported perforation rates. The rates are not necessarily representative of those for any type of IUD. Cervical perforations are not included in this appendix. The uterine perforation rates are primarily for interval IUD insertions (i.e., for insertions performed at least six weeks after a delivery or at least one month after an abortion). Some studies, however, may have included some postpartum and postabortal insertions.

Reference Number	IUD	Number of Insertions	Perforations Number	Rate/1000 Insertions
8	Birnberg Bow	1,045	16	15.3
	Lippes Loop	1,871	2	1.1
	Nylon Ring	225	0	0.0
	Saf-T-Coil	363	0	0.0
	Stainless Steel Ring	484	1	2.1
9	Lippes Loop	2,696	0	0.0
	Margulies Spiral	510	2	3.9
3	Birnberg Bow	544	16	29.4
	Lippes Loop	751	2	2.7
15	Birnberg Bow	169	0	0.0
	Lippes Loop	1,503	13	8.6
	Saf-T-Coil	875	0	0.0
11	Dalkon Shield	10,488	25	2.4
	Lippes Loop	6,149	3	0.5
2	Dalkon Shield	803	3	3.7
	Lippes Loop	1,931	8	4.1
	M	274	1	3.6
4	Cu-T	1,153	1	0.9
	Cu-7	1,156	3	2.6

Reference Number	IUD	Perforations		
		Number of Insertions	Number	Rate/1000 Insertions
10	Antigon	884	0	0.0
	Cu-T	939	0	0.0
	Ypsilon	910	0	0.0
18	Margulies Spiral	699	1	1.4
12	Birnberg Bow	585	5	8.5
1	Lippes Loop	2,018	0	0.0
7	Antigon	1,480	0	0.0
14	Dalkon Shield	2,181	0	0.0
13	Cu-7	1,151	1	0.9
17	Ypsilon	2,180	0	0.0
5	Lippes Loop	6,872	12	1.7
6	Saf-T-Coil	2,952	0	0.0
16	Cu-T	1,531	0	0.0

References

1. Arumugan, L. G. History of contraception and introduction of intra-uterine contraceptive devices in a rural area—Bandaragama, Ceylon. *Acta Obstet. Gynecol.* (Scand) 48:550, 1969.

2. Boria, M. C., and Gordon, M. What to expect when you insert an I.U.D. *Medical Times* 103:93, 1975.

3. Buchman, M. I. A study of the intrauterine contraceptive device with and without an extracervical appendage or tail. *Fertil. Steril.* 21:348, 1970.

4. Cederqvist, L. L.; Lindhe, B-A.; and Fuchs, F. Perforation of the uterus by the Copper-T and Copper-7 intrauterine contraceptive devices. *Acta Obstet. Gynecol.* (Scand) 54:183, 1975.

5. Family Planning Research Unit. *General assessment of the Lippes Loop intrauterine device,* report no. 19.

Exeter: Family Planning Research Unit. University of Exeter, 1977.

6. Family Planning Research Unit. *General assessment of the Saf-T-Coil intrauterine device,* report no. 20. Exeter: Family Planning Research Unit, University of Exeter, 1977.

7. Fuchs, F., and Risk, A. The Antigon-F, an improved intrauterine contraceptive device. *Contraception* 5: 119, 1972.

8. Hall, R. A reappraisal of intrauterine contraceptive devices. Prompted by the discovery of uterine perforations. *Am. J. Obstet. Gynecol.* 99:808, 1967.

9. Kushner, D. H.; Jaffurs, W. J.; Townsend, C. E.; and Thomas, M. A. Surgical and obstetrical complications of intrauterine devices in a specialty hospital. *Int. J. Fertil.* 14:48, 1969.

10. Lauersen, N. H.; Cederqvist, L. L.; Donovan, S.; and Fuchs, F. Comparison of three intrauterine contraceptive devices: the Antigon-F, the Ypsilon-Y, and the Copper-T 200. *Fertil. Steril.* 26:638, 1975.

11. Ma, H. K.; Wei, M.; and Luk, K. F. The Hong Kong experience in the use of the Dalkon Shield. *Contraception* 10:113, 1974.

12. Nakamoto, M., and Buchman, M. I. Complications of intrauterine contraceptive devices: report of 5 cases of ectopic placement of the Bow. *Am. J. Obstet. Gynecol.* 94:1073, 1966.

13. Newton, J.; Elias, J.; McEwan, J.; and Mann, G. Intra-uterine contraception with the Copper 7: evaluation after two years. *Br. Med. J.* 3:447, 1974.

14. Ostergard, D. R., and Broen, E. M. The insertion of intrauterine devices by physicians and paramedical personnel. *Obstet. Gynecol.* 41:257, 1973.

15. Portnuff. J. C.; Ballon, S. C.; and Langer, A. The intra-uterine contraceptive device. A prospective 5 year clinical study. *Am. J. Obstet. Gynecol.* 114:934, 1972.

16. Prema, K., and Phillips, F. S. Long term use of Cu-T 200. Abstract in *Proceedings of the First Asian Congress of Fertility and Sterility*, February 19–23, 1977, Bombay, India.

17. Soichet, S.; Rodrigues, S.; and Cederqvist, L. Experience with a modified small size Ypsilon. *Adv. Plann. Parent.* X:16, 1975.

18. Willson, J. R.; Ledger, W. J.; Bollinger, C. C.; and Andros, G. J. The Margulies intrauterine contraceptive device. Experience with 623 women. *Am. J. Obstet. Gynecol.* 92:63, 1965.

Appendix B

Case-Control Studies, the Odds
Ratio and Relative Risk

Case-control studies, the odds ratio and relative risk are described in terms of a study conducted to assess the association between IUD use and PID. In the case-control study, a group of women with PID (cases) and a group of women without PID (controls) are selected. One or more controls may be matched on the basis of relevant variables to each case. The matching variables might include some or all of the following: age, parity, marital status, time since last pregnancy and prior history of PID. In the selection of the cases only women who are at risk of using an IUD are selected (e.g., women aged 15–44). The selection of cases or controls is not made on the basis of their contraceptive practice, except that women are excluded if they have been sterilized, or are otherwise not at risk of using an IUD.

The data resulting from the selection of cases and controls can be displayed as follows:

	IUD User		
	Yes (A)	No ($\overline{A}$)	Total
Women with PID (B)	n_{11}	n_{12}	n_1
Women Without PID ($\overline{B}$)	n_{21}	n_{22}	n_2
Total	$n_{.1}$	$n_{.2}$	$n_{.1}$

If the cases and controls have not been matched, the odds ratio, 0, is given by:

$$0 = \frac{\text{Odds that an IUD user will have PID}}{\text{Odds that a nonuser will have PID}}$$

$$= \frac{P(B|A) / P(\overline{B}|A)}{P(B|\overline{A}) / P(\overline{B}|\overline{A})}$$

The symbol $P(X|Y)$ is used to denote the probability of event X occurring given that event Y has occurred. The

245

event, B, denotes a woman has PID, and, $\overline{B}$, a woman does not have PID. The event A denotes an IUD user and $\overline{A}$, a nonuser.

It can be shown that the following expression for 0 is equivalent to the above one:

$$\frac{P(A|B) / P(\overline{A}|B)}{P(A|\overline{B}) / P(\overline{A}|\overline{B})} \text{ where}$$

$$P(A|\overline{B}) = n_{11}/n_{1.}, P(\overline{A}|B) = n_{12}/n_{1.},$$

$$P(A|B) = n_{21}/n_{2.}, P(\overline{A}|\overline{B}) = n_{22}/n_{2.}, \text{ and}$$

$$0 = \frac{(n_{11}/n_{1.}) / (n_{12}/n_{1.})}{(n_{21}/n_{2.}) / (n_{22}/n_{2.})} = \frac{n_{11}n_{22}}{n_{21}n_{12}}$$

The probabilities of having or not having PID given the woman is or is not an IUD user [$P(B|A)$, $P(B|\overline{A})$, $P(\overline{B}|A)$ and $P(\overline{B}|\overline{A})$] cannot be estimated from the case-control study data, since only a sample of women with PID and a sample of women without PID were selected. However, the probabilities of being or not being an IUD user given the woman does or does not have PID [$P(A|B)$, $P(\overline{A}|B)$, $P(A|\overline{B})$ and $P(\overline{A}|\overline{B})$] can be estimated from the case-control study data. In a prospective study in which two cohorts of women (IUD users and nonusers) are observed, one can estimate the probabilities $P(B|A)$, $P(\overline{B}|A)$, $P(B|\overline{A})$ and $P(\overline{B}|\overline{A})$.

The relative risk, RR, of the occurrence of PID among IUD users to the occurrence of PID among nonusers is given by:

$$RR = \frac{P(B|A)}{P(B|\overline{A})}$$

In a prospective study if the event B (PID) is unlikely whether or not characteristic A (IUD use) is present, then RR approximates 0, the odds ratio.

In studies where controls are matched to cases, the odds ratio is computed as the ratio of the number of matched pairs of women in which the case is an IUD user, and the control is not, to the number of matched pairs of women in which the case is not an IUD user and the control is an IUD user.

An approximate two-sided $100(1-\alpha)\%$ confidence interval estimate on the odds ratio (1) is given by:

$$\exp [\hat{O} \pm Z_{1-\alpha/2} (SE(\hat{O}))]$$

where: $\hat{O}$ is the estimated odds ratio.

$Z_{1-\alpha/2}$ is the 100 $(1-\alpha/2)$ percentile point of the standard normal distribution.
$SE(\hat{O})$ is the standard error of $\hat{O}$ and is estimated from the relationship $[\ln_e \hat{O}/SE(0)]^2 = \chi^2$, where χ^2 is the chi-square statistic computed from a 2×2 table.

Neither the odds ratio nor relative risk provides a measure of the increased risk of PID attributable to IUD use among IUD users compared to nonusers. Such a measure of attributable risk (AR) can be calculated in a cohort study as the difference in the rates of PID among IUD users and nonusers:

$$AR = P(B|A) - P(B|\overline{A})$$

Reference

1. Miettinem, O. Simple interval-estimation of risk ratio. *Am. J. Epid.* 100:515, 1974.

Appendix C

Listed in this appendix are a selected group of studies which have reported on PID in association with IUD use. The studies are not necessarily representative of all studies, but they were selected to illustrate the range of PID rates and IUD removals for PID as reported by different investigators.

Reference Number	IUD	Number of Insertions	Removals for PID Number	Removals for PID Percentage	All Cases of PID Number	All Cases of PID Percentage
5	Birnberg Bow	885	—	—	21	2.4
	Lippes Loop	788	—	—	14	1.8
	Saf-T-Coil	347	—	—	19	5.5
	Nylon Ring	33	—	—	1	3.0
	Steel Ring	277	—	—	6	2.2
3	Birnberg Bow	128	—	—	1	0.8
	Lippes Loop	149	—	—	27	18.1
1	Birnberg Bow	544	12	2.2	19	3.5
	Lippes Loop	751	—	—	6	0.8
11	Birnberg Bow	169	—	—	2	1.2
	Lippes Loop	1,503	—	—	16	1.1
	Saf-T-Coil	875	—	—	9	1.0
2	Dalkon Shield	206	1	0.5	—	—
	Lippes Loop	209	2	1.0	—	—
	Cu-T-300	361	2	0.6	—	—
13	Dalkon Shield	4,677	21	0.5	28	0.6
	Lippes Loop	4,447	5	0.1	10	0.2
	Saf-T-Coil	1,613	3	0.2	3	0.2
	Cu-7	3,700	17	0.5	24	0.6
14	Dalkon Shield	347	—	—	11	3.2
	Cu-T	668	—	—	9	1.3
15	Lippes Loop	750	6	0.8	—	—
	Cu-T	945	8	0.8	—	—
20	Margulies Spiral	623	8	1.3	48	7.7

Reference Number	IUD	Number of Insertions	Removals for PID Number	Removals for PID Percentage	All Cases of PID Number	All Cases of PID Percentage
8	Birnberg Bow	339	7	2.1	31	9.1
19	Lippes Loop	710	8	1.1	11	1.5
4	Dalkon Shield	1,303	36	2.8	44	3.4
16	Majzlin Spring	410	33	8.0	—	—
7	Dalkon Shield	2,007	0	0.0	1	0.1
9	Cu-7	1,156	2	0.2	—	—
6	Cu-7	281	9	3.2	—	—
12	Ypsilon	2,180	14	0.6	—	—
18	Cu-T	3,016	—	—	90	3.0
10	Cu-T	750	—	—	16	2.1
17	Cu-T/Cu-7	243	7	2.9	—	—

References

1. Buchman, M. I. A study of the intrauterine contraceptive device with and without an extracervical appendage or tail. *Fertil. Steril.* 21:348, 1970.

2. Cooper, D. L.; Israel, R.; and Mishell, D. R. Randomized comparative study of the Copper T 300, Dalkon Shield, and Shell Loop in parous women. *Obstet. Gynecol.* 45:569, 1975.

3. Elstein, M. Pelvic inflammation and the intrauterine contraceptive device. *Proc. Roy. Soc. Med.* 60:397, 1969.

4. Gabrielson, M. O.; Goldsmith, S.; and Stangeland, S. Dalkon Shield and the young nulliparous patient: eighteen months' experience. *Adv. Plann. Parent.* 8: 138, 1973.

5. Hall, R. E. A comparative evaluation of intrauterine contraceptive devices. *Am. J. Obstet. Gynecol.* 94: 65, 1966.

6. Houghton, H. An analysis of 649 patients attending a family planning clinic. *J. Fam. Plann. Doctors* 1:13, 1975.

7. Ma, H. K.; Wei, M.; and Luk, K. F. The Hong Kong experience in the use of the Dalkon Shield. *Contraception* 10:113, 1974.

8. McCammon, R. The Birnberg Bow as an intrauterine contraceptive device. *Obstet. Gynecol.* 29:67, 1967.

9. Newton, J.; Elias, J.; McEwan, J.; and Mann, G. Intrauterine contraception with the Copper 7: evaluation after two years. *Br. Med. J.* 3:447, 1974.

10. Osser, S.; Gullberg, B.; Liedholm, P.; and Sjoberg, N-O. Is development of pelvic inflammatory disease in women using intrauterine device equal regardless of parity? A one year follow-up study. *Contraception* 17:563, 1978.

11. Portnuff, J. C.; Ballon, S. L.; and Langer, A. The intrauterine contraceptive device. A prospective 5 year clinical study. *Am. J. Obstet Gynecol.* 114:934, 1972.

12. Rodrigues, W.; and Nogueira, T. A study of the Ypsilon IUD in Brazil. *Adv. Plann. Parent.* X:221, 1975.

13. Snowden, R. Pelvic inflammation, perforation, and pregnancy outcome associated with the use of IUDs. In *Analysis of intrauterine contraception*, eds. F. Hefnawi and S. J. Segal. New York: American Elsevier Publishing Co., Inc., 1975.

14. Spellacy, W. N.; Birk, S. A.; and Gordon, L. Comparative randomized study of the Copper-T 200 and Dalkon Shield intrauterine devices. *Contraception* 12:453, 1975.

15. Tatum, H. The first year of clinical experience with the Copper T intrauterine contraceptive system in the United States and Canada. *Adv. Plann. Parent.* 8:127, 1973.

16. Taylor, W. W.; Martin, F. G.; Pritchard, S. A.; and Pritchard, J. A. Complications from Majzlin Spring intrauterine device. *Obstet. Gynecol.* 41:404, 1973.

17. Weiner, E.; Berg, A. A.; and Johansson, I. Copper intrauterine contraceptive devices in adolescent nulliparae. *Brit. J. Obstet. Gynaecol.* 85:204, 1978.

18. Williamson, H. O.; Bank, H. L.; Kirkland, B. H.; and Tatum, T. Experience with 3000 patients. *Adv. Plann. Parent.* X:95, 1975.

19. Willson, J. R., and Ledger, W. J. Complications associated with the use of intrauterine contraceptive devices in women of middle and upper socioeconomic class. *Am. J. Obstet. Gynecol.* 100:649, 1968.

20. Willson, J. R.; Ledger, W. J.; Bollinger, C. C.; and Andros, G. J. The Margulies intrauterine contraceptive device. Experience with 623 women. *Am. J. Obstet. Gynecol.* 92:62, 1965.

Index

postinsertion pain of, 44
postpartum expulsion rates for,
40
and pregnancy rates, 30
retention of, 124
return to fertility after use of,
224
spontaneous abortion associated
with, 174, 177, 178
uterine perforations associated
with, 244
Copper-T IUD, 7, 8, 10
bacteriologic studies on, 95
bowel perforation associated
with, 73
and cervical neoplasia, 165
cervical perforation rates for, 58,
70
congenital abnormalities associated with, 186
ectopic pregnancy associated
with, 205, 208
ectopic pregnancy rates (EPR)
for, 206
fibrinolytic activity associated
with, 148
and gonorrheal infections, 99,
100
and hospitalization for PID, 117
insertion of, 70
insertion difficulties with, 43
intrauterine pregnancy associated with, 176
laparoscopic removal of, 76, 77
menstrual blood loss associated
with, 141, 142, 143, 144, 145,
146
ovarian pregnancy associated
with, 207
perforations incidence for, 57
perforation rates for, 56
PID associated with, 105, 248,
249
PID rates for, 111, 119
postabortal insertion of, 38, 39
and postinsertion changes in
vital signs, 45
postinsertion pain of, 44
postpartum expulsion rates for,
40
pregnancy and expulsion rates

associated with, 15
retention of, 124
return to fertility after use of,
224
spontaneous abortion associated
with, 177, 178
timing of insertion of, 36
tubo-ovarian abscesses associated with, 121, 122
uterine perforations associated
with, 244
uterine perforation rates for, 77
Copper wire, 8
Coralle IUD, 7
Cramping, associated with IUD insertion, 43. See also Pain
CSP. See Cooperative Statistical
Program
Cuivre IUD, 7
Culdocentesis, 203
Curettage, 152
Cu-7. See Copper-7 IUD
Cu-T. See Copper-T IUD

Dalkon Shield, 7
abdominal pregnancy as-
sociated with, 207
abdominopelvic adhesions associated with, 75
actinomycosis infections associated with, 123
bladder perforation associated
with, 73
bowel perforation associated
with, 73
cervical perforation rates for, 70
chronic salpingitis associated
with, 109
complicated pregnancy as-
sociated with, 115, 180
congenital abnormalities associated with, 185
continuation rates for, 238
deaths associated with, 179
ectopic pregnancy associated
with, 205
and fibrinolytic activity, 149
grand mal seizures associated
with, 46
hospitalizations associated
with, 58, 115, 117, 180

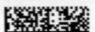